THIS GUIDED JOURNAL BELONGS TO

feelings journal pages

feelings tool kit

practice pages

The Feelings Wheel was created by Dr. Gloria Willcox in 1982 to aid people in learning to recognize and communicate about their feelings.

Feelings Pie
A Guided Journal Through The Feelings Wheel

FeelingsPie.com
BlueIguanaEducation.com

ISBN: 979-8-218-36200-3

Welcome to Feelings Pie!

As you begin this journey of self-exploration, try to be kind and nonjudgemental with yourself. Keep in mind that there is no such thing as a "good" or "bad" feeling. All of them are okay to have, and any feeling you experience is valid. Use this guided journal to help you navigate through your feelings and understand yourself better.

There are many different approaches to using Feelings Pie and you get to decide which path you prefer. You might begin at the heart of a core feeling, expanding outward to explore some of the more specific feelings. Or you could choose to dive into a random page, letting chance guide your exploration. Another option would be to chronicle your feelings in real time, capturing the experience of each feeling as it arises in your day-to-day life. There is no prescribed method to navigate through these pages. This journey is uniquely yours, and you hold the reins.

Within the Feelings Tool Kit, you'll find resources to help you dig a little deeper as you walk this path of self-discovery. In doing so, please keep in mind that seeking support is a sign of strength. If you encounter challenging or overwhelming feelings while working through these pages, we encourage you to seek the help of a licensed mental health professional. They can offer individualized support and guidance on your journey and shine a light when you need it the most.

As you work through Feelings Pie, pause to acknowledge that you are inherently complete and perfect as you are. Your feelings, thoughts, and experiences make you uniquely you. Take this opportunity to practice gentle self-acceptance and self-love as you deepen your understanding of your inner world. And then use what you learn here to enhance your relationship with yourself and with others.

Wishing you all the best on your self-discovery journey!

How to Use The Feelings Wheel

The Feelings Wheel is like a colorful map that helps you discover and understand your feelings. Here's how to use it:

Look at the Colors and Words: The wheel is full of colors and words that represent feelings. The very center has core feelings like happy, sad, scared, or angry. As you move outward, the feelings get more specific.

Identify Your Core Feeling: Start at the center of the wheel. Are you feeling happy, sad, scared, or angry right now? Pick the one that most closely matches how you feel.

Explore More Specific Feelings: Once you've identified your core feeling, move to the outer circles. They have more feelings that are related to the one you identified. For example, if you chose "happy" in the inner circle, the outer circles have feelings like "content", "excited", and "curious".

Understand Your Exact Feeling: Explore the more detailed and specific feelings of the outer circles to see which ones seem to fit. Try on a few for size until you begin to understand exactly how you're feeling. For instance, if you started with "peaceful" you might realize you actually feel "trusting" or "loving".

Talk About It: Now that you know how you feel, you can talk about it with someone you trust, like a friend, family member or therapist. Understanding your feelings makes it easier to explain them to others.

Use It Regularly: The Feelings Wheel is a tool you can use anytime you're not sure about how you are feeling. The more you use it, the better you'll get at identifying and understanding your feelings.

Remember, every feeling on the wheel is okay to have. There is no such thing as a "good" or "bad" feeling. All of them are okay to have, and any feeling you experience is valid. Use the Feelings Wheel as a guide to help you navigate through your feelings and understand yourself better. Just like a detective uses clues to solve a mystery, you can use the Feelings Wheel to figure out your feelings.

The Feelings Wheel

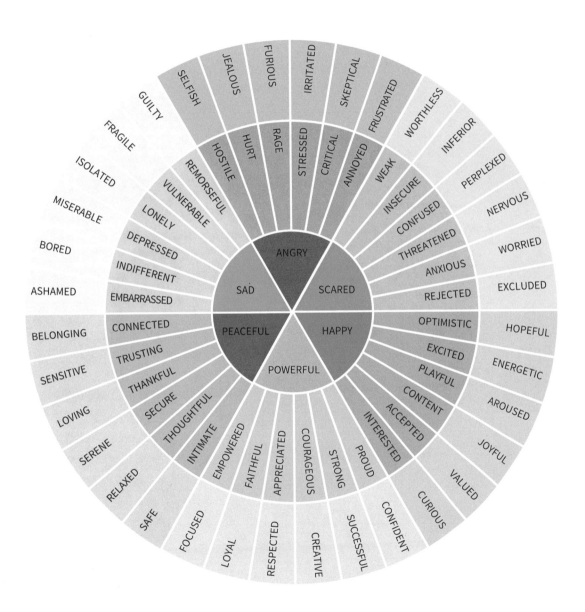

FEELINGS
JOURNAL
PAGES

GUILTY
FRAGILE
SH
HOSTILE
REMORSE
HURT
RAGE
STRESSED
CRITICAL
ANNOYED
SK
FRUSTRA
WORTHLESS
INFERIOR
PERPLEX
WEAK
SECURE
ATED
VULNERABLE
LONELY
CONFUSED
NE
LE
DEPRESSED
THREATENED
INDIFFERENT
ANXIOUS
EMBARRASSED
REJECTED
CONNECTED
PEACEFUL
HAPPY
OPTIMISTIC
TRUSTING
EXCITED
THANKFUL
POWERFUL
PLAYFUL
E
SECURE
THOUGHTFUL
CONTENT
AR
INTIMATE
EMPOWERED
FAITHFUL
APPRECIATED
COURAGEOUS
STRONG
PROUD
INTERESTED
ACCEPTED
RENE
JOYFU
RELAXED
VALUED
SAFE
FOCUSED
LOYAL
RESPECTED
CREATIVE
SUCCESSFUL
CONFIDENT
CURIOUS

Happy

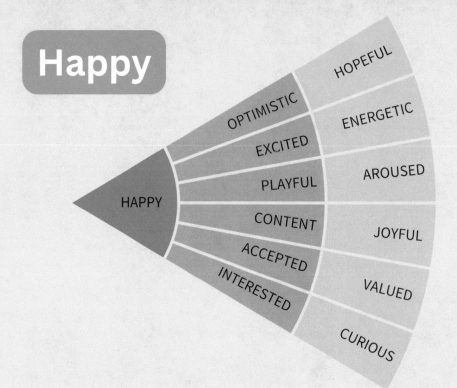

OPTIMISTIC
HOPEFUL
EXCITED
ENERGETIC
PLAYFUL
AROUSED
HAPPY
CONTENT
JOYFUL
ACCEPTED
INTERESTED
VALUED
CURIOUS

These are some of the feelings in the happy group. Sometimes when people experience feelings in the happy group they exhibit the following behaviors:

- Smiling or laughing
- Engaging in social interaction
- Expressing gratitude
- Showing a high level of energy
- Being more generous or helpful
- Displaying relaxed body language
- Being talkative and sharing positive stories
- Demonstrating patience and tolerance
- Singing or humming to themself
- Initiating contact or closeness with others

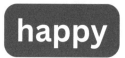

happy

enjoying pleasure, satisfaction and contentment

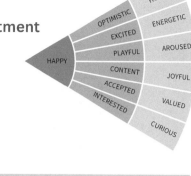

Sometimes people feel happy when:

- They receive good news
- Celebrating a special occasion with loved ones
- They accomplish a personal goal
- Spending time engaged in a favorite hobby

I feel happy when...

One recent time I felt happy was...

When that happened I expressed myself by...

Other ways I have expressed happiness are...

When I express happiness it impacts the people around me by...

Next time I feel happy I would like to...

By exploring how I feel and express happiness I have learned about myself...

optimistic

hopeful about the future and confident that positive outcomes are likely

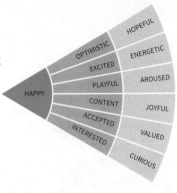

Sometimes people feel optimistic when:

- They receive positive feedback from a teacher
- Starting a new and exciting project
- The weather forecast for an event looks good
- They read encouraging news

I feel optimistic when...

One recent time I felt optimistic was...

When that happened I expressed myself by...

Other ways I have expressed optimism are...

When I express optimism it impacts the people around me by...

Next time I feel optimistic I would like to...

By exploring how I feel and express optimism I have learned about myself...

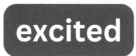

excited

enthusiastic and eager

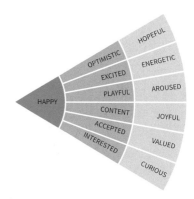

Sometimes people feel excited when:

- They are planning a vacation
- Receiving a gift they have wanted for a long time
- Anticipating a visit from a close friend
- They have won a contest

I feel excited when...

One recent time I felt excited was...   **When that happened I expressed myself by...**

Other ways I have expressed excitement are...

When I express excitement it impacts the people around me by...   **Next time I feel excited I would like to...**

By exploring how I feel and express excitement I have learned about myself...

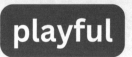

playful

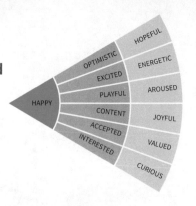

inclined to play and engage in lighthearted activities; fun-loving

Sometimes people feel playful when:

- They are joking with or poking fun at their partner
- Trying out a new board game with friends
- They play with a new pet at home
- Building a sandcastle on the beach

I feel playful when...

One recent time I felt playful was...

When that happened I expressed myself by...

Other ways I have expressed playfulness are...

When I express playfulness it impacts the people around me by...

Next time I feel playful I would like to...

By exploring how I feel and express playfulness I have learned about myself...

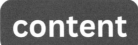

content

satisfied and at ease with one's current situation

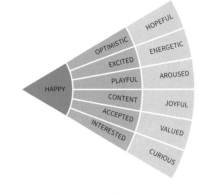

Sometimes people feel content when:

- They enjoy a quiet evening at home with a good book
- Finding comfort in a daily routine
- They have a hearty meal with family
- Taking a moment to appreciate a beautiful sunset

I feel content when...

One recent time I felt content was...

When that happened I expressed myself by...

Other ways I have expressed contentment are...

When I express contentment it impacts the people around me by...

Next time I feel content I would like to...

By exploring how I feel and express contentment I have learned about myself...

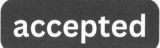

accepted

received or treated as adequate or suitable

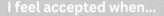

Sometimes people feel accepted when:

- Being included in a new social circle
- Receiving affirmation from peers
- Being welcomed into a new neighborhood
- They are unconditionally supported by their family

I feel accepted when...

One recent time I felt accepted was...

When that happened I expressed myself by...

Other ways I have expressed acceptance are...

When I express acceptance it impacts the people around me by...

Next time I feel accepted I would like to...

By exploring how I feel and express acceptance I have learned about myself...

interested

showing curiosity or concern about something or someone; eager to learn more

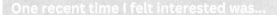

Sometimes people feel interested when:

- They discover a new hobby
- Watching a documentary on a favorite subject
- They engage in conversation that sparks curiosity
- Listening to new music from a favorite band

I feel interested when...

One recent time I felt interested was...

When that happened I expressed myself by...

Other ways I have expressed interest are...

When I express interest it impacts the people around me by...

Next time I feel interested I would like to...

By exploring how I feel and express interest I have learned about myself...

hopeful

optimistic that what is desired may happen and all will turn out for the best

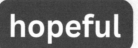

Sometimes people feel hopeful when:

- Waiting to see if seeds will grow into flowers
- Looking forward to a fun new class
- They audition for a team or community play
- Aspiring to see change after voting in an election

I feel hopeful when...

One recent time I felt hopeful was...

When that happened I expressed myself by...

Other ways I have expressed hopefulness are...

When I express hopefulness it impacts the people around me by...

Next time I feel hopeful I would like to...

By exploring how I feel and express hopefulness I have learned about myself...

energetic

having or showing vitality and enthusiasm; able to exert energy for activities

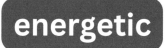

Sometimes people feel energetic when:

- Waking up refreshed after a good night's sleep
- Invigorated after a challenging workout
- Being eager to start a new passion project
- They dance at a concert or music festival

I feel energetic when...

One recent time I felt energetic was...   When that happened I expressed myself by...

Other ways I have expressed energy are...

When I express energy it impacts the people around me by...   Next time I feel energetic I would like to...

By exploring how I feel and express energy I have learned about myself...

aroused

stirred up to a strong response, into a state of heightened energy or activity

Sometimes people feel aroused when:

- They are about to enter a competition or race
- Experiencing a burst of motivation
- Their interest is piqued by an upcoming movie
- Experiencing a stimulating art exhibit

I feel aroused when...

One recent time I felt aroused was...

When that happened I expressed myself by...

Other ways I have expressed arousal are...

When I express arousal it impacts the people around me by...

Next time I feel aroused I would like to...

By exploring how I feel and express arousal I have learned about myself...

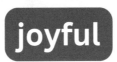

joyful

experiencing great happiness,
pleasure and delight

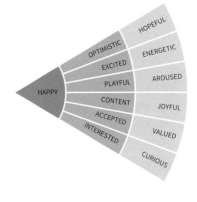

Sometimes people feel joyful when:

- Celebrating a significant personal achievement
- They hear good news about a loved one's health
- Watching a favorite sports team win a game
- They spend an evening engaged in a favorite activity

I feel joyful when...

One recent time I felt joyful was...

When that happened I expressed myself by...

Other ways I have expressed joyfulness are...

When I express joyfulness it impacts the people around me by...

Next time I feel joyful I would like to...

By exploring how I feel and express joyfulness I have learned about myself...

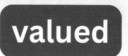

valued

appreciated and held in high regard

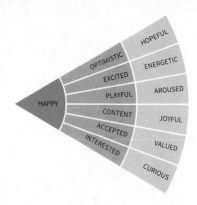

Sometimes people feel valued when:

- Receiving recognition for their contributions
- Being thanked sincerely for helping a friend
- Their advice is sought after by a peer
- Knowing they are an important part of a team

I feel valued when...

One recent time I felt valued was...

When that happened I expressed myself by...

Other ways I have expressed value are...

When I express value it impacts the people around me by...

Next time I feel valued I would like to...

By exploring how I feel and express value I have learned about myself...

curious

eager to know or learn something; having a strong desire for understanding or knowledge

Sometimes people feel curious when:

- Exploring a new city while on vacation
- They read a great mystery novel
- Trying out a new cuisine
- Asking questions about a friend's unusual hobby

I feel curious when...

One recent time I felt curious was...

When that happened I expressed myself by...

Other ways I have expressed curiosity are...

When I express curiosity it impacts the people around me by...

Next time I feel curious I would like to...

By exploring how I feel and express curiosity I have learned about myself...

summary and reflection

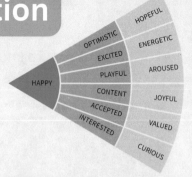

Which feeling was the easiest to write about? Why do you think that is?

Which feeling did you have the most examples for?

Which feeling was the most difficult to write about? Why do you think that is?

Which feeling was the hardest to identify?

What surprised you while journaling about your happy feelings?

Did journaling about any of these feelings cause you to feel another feeling?

What have you learned about yourself by journaling about your happy feelings?

Powerful

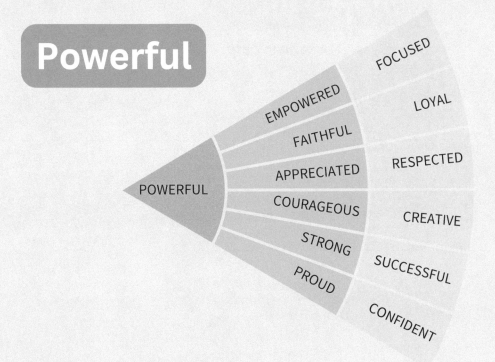

POWERFUL

EMPOWERED
FAITHFUL
APPRECIATED
COURAGEOUS
STRONG
PROUD

FOCUSED
LOYAL
RESPECTED
CREATIVE
SUCCESSFUL
CONFIDENT

These are some of the feelings in the powerful group. Sometimes when people experience feelings in the powerful group they exhibit the following behaviors:

- Taking initiative and leading actions
- Speaking assertively and confidently
- Standing tall with an open posture
- Making decisive choices
- Demonstrating enthusiasm in their pursuits
- Offering opinions and advice
- Taking on responsibilities willingly
- Encouraging or motivating others
- Persisting in the face of setbacks
- Celebrating successes openly

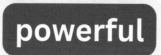

powerful

confident, capable and in control

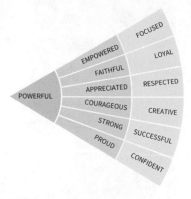

Sometimes people feel powerful when:

- They achieve a significant accomplishment
- Exercising leadership or influence
- They overcome a difficult challenge
- Mastering a new skill or knowledge area

I feel powerful when...

One recent time I felt powerful was...

When that happened I expressed myself by...

Other ways I have expressed powerfulness are...

When I express powerfulness it impacts the people around me by...

Next time I feel powerful I would like to...

By exploring how I feel and express powerfulness I have learned about myself...

empowered

confidence in one's abilities and
in control of one's life

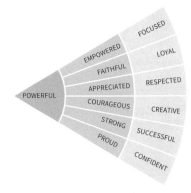

Sometimes people feel empowered when:

- Successfully advocating for a cause
- They learn a new skill
- Overcoming a personal fear or challenge
- They make a significant life decision

I feel empowered when...

One recent time I felt empowered was...   **When that happened I expressed myself by...**

Other ways I have expressed empowerment are...

When I express empowerment it impacts the people around me by...   **Next time I feel empowered I would like to...**

By exploring how I feel and express empowerment I have learned about myself...

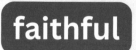

faithful

true to one's word, promises or vows;
steady in allegiance or affection

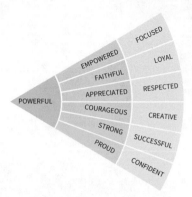

Sometimes people feel faithful when:

- Maintaining a long-term commitment to a partner
- They uphold a promise made to a friend
- Sticking to their values despite external pressures
- They practice religious or spiritual beliefs

I feel faithful when...

One recent time I felt faithful was...

When that happened I expressed myself by...

Other ways I have expressed faithfulness are...

When I express faithfulness it impacts the people around me by...

Next time I feel faithful I would like to...

By exploring how I feel and express faithfulness I have learned about myself...

appreciated

**highly valued or esteemed;
regarded with thankfulness**

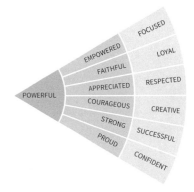

Sometimes people feel appreciated when:

- They receive a thank-you note for helping someone
- Being acknowledged for hard work on a project
- Receiving thanks from a partner for doing chores
- They are credited for their ideas

I feel appreciated when...

One recent time I felt appreciated was...   **When that happened I expressed myself by...**

Other ways I have expressed appreciation are...

When I express appreciation it impacts the people around me by...   **Next time I feel appreciated I would like to...**

By exploring how I feel and express appreciation I have learned about myself...

courageous

being brave; facing fear or challenges head-on

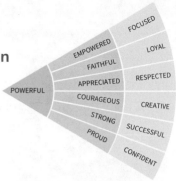

Sometimes people feel courageous when:

- Speaking up against injustice despite personal risk
- They try something new despite the fear of failure
- They stand up for someone who is being bullied
- Tackling a challenging outdoor adventure sport

I feel courageous when...

One recent time I felt courageous was...   **When that happened I expressed myself by...**

Other ways I have expressed courageousness are...

When I express courageousness it impacts the people around me by...   **Next time I feel courageous I would like to...**

By exploring how I feel and express courageousness I have learned about myself...

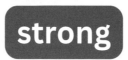

strong

difficult to break, destroy, or make sick;
able to support a heavy weight

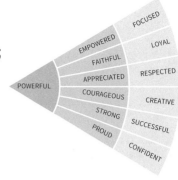

Sometimes people feel strong when:

- They overcome a difficult challenge
- Persisting through a tough task until completion
- They support a friend through struggles
- Recovering from an illness or injury with resilience

I feel strong when...

One recent time I felt strong was...

When that happened I expressed myself by...

Other ways I have expressed strength are...

When I express strength it impacts the people around me by...

Next time I feel strong I would like to...

By exploring how I feel and express strength I have learned about myself...

proud

a deep sense of satisfaction from one's own or another's achievements

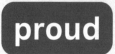

FOCUSED
EMPOWERED
LOYAL
FAITHFUL
APPRECIATED
RESPECTED
POWERFUL
COURAGEOUS
CREATIVE
STRONG
SUCCESSFUL
PROUD
CONFIDENT

Sometimes people feel proud when:

- Being acknowledged for their role in a project
- Their artwork is displayed in a public space
- They receive a personal compliment from a peer
- Reflecting on their personal growth & development

I feel proud when...

One recent time I felt proud was...

When that happened I expressed myself by...

Other ways I have expressed pride are...

When I express pride it impacts the people around me by...

Next time I feel proud I would like to...

By exploring how I feel and express pride I have learned about myself...

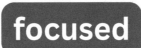

focused

clear perception or understanding;
directed attention

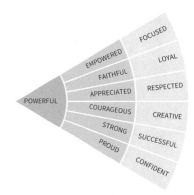

Sometimes people feel focused when:

- They work intently on a project until it is complete
- Studying for an important exam
- They practice playing a challenging piece of music
- Engaging in a meditative or spiritual practice

I feel focused when...

One recent time I felt focused was...

When that happened I expressed myself by...

Other ways I have expressed focus are...

When I express focus it impacts the people around me by...

Next time I feel focused I would like to...

By exploring how I feel and express focus I have learned about myself...

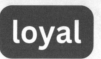

loyal

showing strong support or allegiance to someone or something

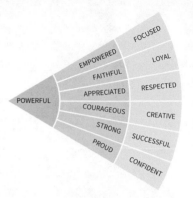

Sometimes people feel loyal when:

- They stand by a friend during difficult times
- Showing unwavering support to a sports team
- They commit to a relationship through challenges
- Defending a loved one against criticism

I feel loyal when...

One recent time I felt loyal was...

When that happened I expressed myself by...

Other ways I have expressed loyalty are...

When I express loyalty it impacts the people around me by...

Next time I feel loyal I would like to...

By exploring how I feel and express loyalty I have learned about myself...

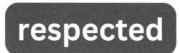

respected

worthy of high regard

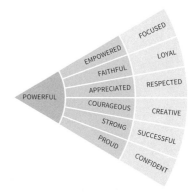

Sometimes people feel respected when:

- Their boundaries are acknowledged and upheld
- Receiving an award for achievements
- Their opinion is sought after in discussions
- Being looked up to by younger family members

I feel respected when...

One recent time I felt respected was...

When that happened I expressed myself by...

Other ways I have expressed respect are...

When I express respect it impacts the people around me by...

Next time I feel respected I would like to...

By exploring how I feel and express respect I have learned about myself...

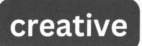
creative

original and expressive in thoughts or actions

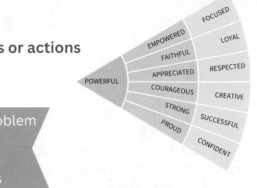

Sometimes people feel creative when:

- Coming up with an innovative solution to a problem
- Starting a new art project and feeling inspired
- They write a piece of music or literature
- Brainstorming a unique concept for a business

I feel creative when...

One recent time I felt creative was...

When that happened I expressed myself by...

Other ways I have expressed creativity are...

When I express creativity it impacts the people around me by...

Next time I feel creative I would like to...

By exploring how I feel and express creativity I have learned about myself...

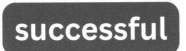

successful

accomplishing an aim or purpose

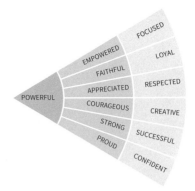

Sometimes people feel successful when:

- Achieving a long-term personal or professional goal
- They complete a marathon or fitness challenge
- Their work is featured or recognized publicly
- Graduating from a program of study

I feel successful when...

One recent time I felt successful was...

When that happened I expressed myself by...

Other ways I have expressed successfulness are...

When I express successfulness it impacts the people around me by...

Next time I feel successful I would like to...

By exploring how I feel and express successfulness I have learned about myself...

confident

having or showing assurance and self-reliance

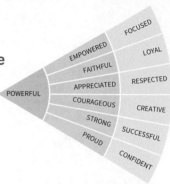

Sometimes people feel confident when:

- Navigating a difficult situation with ease
- They receive compliments on their expertise
- Knowing they are prepared for a competition
- They wear an outfit that makes them feel powerful

I feel confident when...

One recent time I felt confident was...

When that happened I expressed myself by...

Other ways I have expressed confidence are...

When I express confidence it impacts the people around me by...

Next time I feel confident I would like to...

By exploring how I feel and express confidence I have learned about myself...

summary and reflection

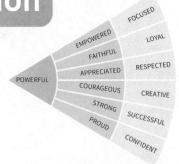

EMPOWERED · FOCUSED · FAITHFUL · LOYAL · APPRECIATED · RESPECTED · POWERFUL · COURAGEOUS · CREATIVE · STRONG · SUCCESSFUL · PROUD · CONFIDENT

Which feeling was the easiest to write about? Why do you think that is?

Which feeling did you have the most examples for?

Which feeling was the most difficult to write about? Why do you think that is?

Which feeling was the hardest to identify?

What surprised you while journaling about your powerful feelings?

Did journaling about any of these feelings cause you to feel another feeling?

What have you learned about yourself by journaling about your powerful feelings?

Peaceful

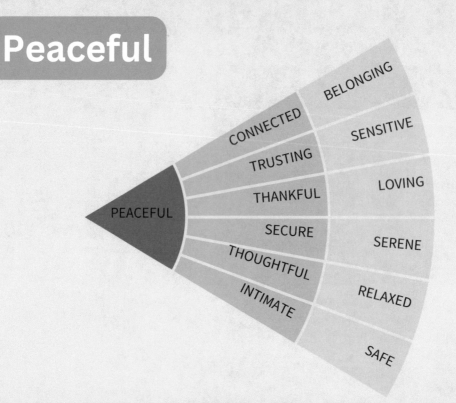

These are some of the feelings in the peaceful group.
Sometimes when people experience feelings in the peaceful group they exhibit the following behaviors:

- Maintaining a calm demeanor
- Speaking in a soft, soothing tone
- Moving gracefully and deliberately
- Showing patience and understanding
- Exhibiting deep, regular breathing
- Offering smiles or gestures of contentment
- Taking time to appreciate their surroundings
- Engaging in leisurely activities
- Demonstrating openness in posture and expression
- Avoiding conflict and seeking harmonious resolutions

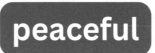
peaceful

untroubled by conflict; tranquil

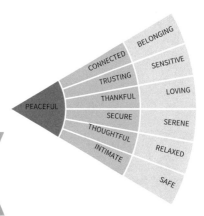

Sometimes people feel peaceful when:

- They practice meditation or yoga
- Being in a natural and serene environment
- There is a sense of harmony in their relationships
- Having a clear conscience by resolving past conflicts

I feel peaceful when...

One recent time I felt peaceful was...   **When that happened I expressed myself by...**

Other ways I have expressed peacefulness are...

When I express peacefulness it impacts the people around me by...   **Next time I feel peaceful I would like to...**

By exploring how I feel and express peacefulness I have learned about myself...

connected

having relationships with others; joined or linked together

Sometimes people feel connected when:

- They have a conversation with a close friend
- Enjoying an inclusive family gathering
- Working harmoniously with a team on a project
- They feel understood and accepted by their partner

PEACEFUL · CONNECTED · TRUSTING · THANKFUL · SECURE · THOUGHTFUL · INTIMATE · BELONGING · SENSITIVE · LOVING · SERENE · RELAXED · SAFE

I feel connected when...

One recent time I felt connected was...

When that happened I expressed myself by...

Other ways I have expressed connection are...

When I express connection it impacts the people around me by...

Next time I feel connected I would like to...

By exploring how I feel and express connection I have learned about myself...

trusting

belief in the character, ability, strength, or truth
of someone or something

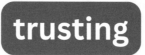

Sometimes people feel trusting when:

- Relying on a friend to keep a significant promise
- They are secure in their partnership
- Believing a doctor's advice is in their best interest
- They have faith that a secret shared will be kept

I feel trusting when...

One recent time I felt trusting was...

When that happened I expressed myself by...

Other ways I have expressed trustfulness are...

When I express trustfulness it impacts the people around me by...

Next time I feel trusting I would like to...

By exploring how I feel and express trustfulness I have learned about myself...

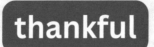

thankful

conscious of benefit received; grateful

CONNECTED BELONGING
TRUSTING SENSITIVE
THANKFUL LOVING
SECURE SERENE
THOUGHTFUL
INTIMATE RELAXED
PEACEFUL
SAFE

Sometimes people feel thankful when:

- A friend is helpful during a difficult time
- Being grateful for good health after an illness
- They have the unwavering support of their family
- They receive a kind gesture from a stranger

I feel thankful when...

One recent time I felt thankful was...

When that happened I expressed myself by...

Other ways I have expressed thankfulness are...

When I express thankfulness it impacts the people around me by...

Next time I feel thankful I would like to...

By exploring how I feel and express thankfulness I have learned about myself...

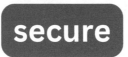

secure

free from danger, fear or anxiety

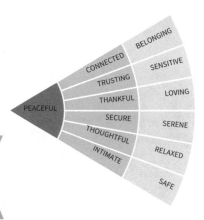

Sometimes people feel secure when:

- They live in a safe and supportive community
- They are emotionally stable and self-assured
- They feel respected by their partner
- They have a reliable job that provides for their needs

I feel secure when...

One recent time I felt secure was...

When that happened I expressed myself by...

Other ways I have expressed security are...

When I express security it impacts the people around me by...

Next time I feel secure I would like to...

By exploring how I feel and express security I have learned about myself...

thoughtful

showing consideration for the needs and feelings of others

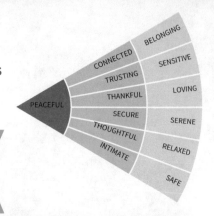

Sometimes people feel thoughtful when:

- They plan a friend's birthday party or anniversary
- They consider the impact of their words & actions
- Doing something helpful without being asked
- Taking time to select a meaningful gift

I feel thoughtful when...

One recent time I felt thoughtful was...

When that happened I expressed myself by...

Other ways I have expressed thoughtfulness are...

When I express thoughtfulness it impacts the people around me by...

Next time I feel thoughtful I would like to...

By exploring how I feel and express thoughtfulness I have learned about myself...

intimate

a close personal association, detailed knowledge
or deep understanding

Sometimes people feel intimate when:

- Having a heart-to-heart talk with a close friend
- They share private moments with a partner
- Bonding with a friend over a shared activity
- They connect with family through shared experiences

CONNECTED
TRUSTING
THANKFUL
SECURE
THOUGHTFUL
INTIMATE
PEACEFUL
BELONGING
SENSITIVE
LOVING
SERENE
RELAXED
SAFE

I feel intimate when...

One recent time I felt intimate was...

When that happened I expressed myself by...

Other ways I have expressed intimacy are...

When I express intimacy it impacts the people around me by...

Next time I feel intimate I would like to...

By exploring how I feel and express intimacy I have learned about myself...

belonging

comfortable and happy in a particular situation or with a particular group of people

Sometimes people feel belonging when:

- They are comfortable in their community
- Being warmly welcomed into a new workplace
- They find people who share their interests
- Receiving acceptance from someone they admire

PEACEFUL
CONNECTED
TRUSTING
THANKFUL
SECURE
THOUGHTFUL
INTIMATE
BELONGING
SENSITIVE
LOVING
SERENE
RELAXED
SAFE

I feel belonging when...

One recent time I felt belonging was...

When that happened I expressed myself by...

Other ways I have expressed belongingness are...

When I express belongingness it impacts the people around me by...

Next time I feel belonging I would like to...

By exploring how I feel and express belongingness I have learned about myself...

sensitive

highly responsive or susceptible to slight changes, signals, or influences

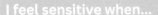

Sometimes people feel sensitive when:

- Noticing a change in a friend's mood
- They are moved by a piece of music or art
- Responding to the subtle needs of a partner
- Feeling touched by a story or character in a book

I feel sensitive when...

One recent time I felt sensitive was...

When that happened I expressed myself by...

Other ways I have expressed sensitivity are...

When I express sensitivity it impacts the people around me by...

Next time I feel sensitive I would like to...

By exploring how I feel and express sensitivity I have learned about myself...

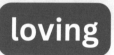

loving

deep affection, warm regard or great care

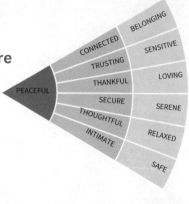

Sometimes people feel loving when:

- They see their pet do something endearing
- Spending quality time with their best friend
- They express affection through words or actions
- Experiencing warmth when their partner is near

I feel loving when...

One recent time I felt loving was...

When that happened I expressed myself by...

Other ways I have expressed lovingness are...

When I express lovingness it impacts the people around me by...

Next time I feel loving I would like to...

By exploring how I feel and express lovingness I have learned about myself...

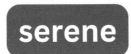

serene

calm, peaceful, and untroubled

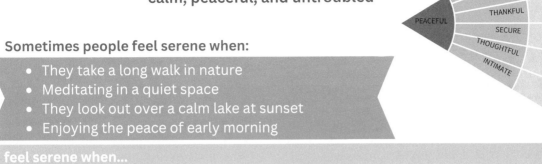

Sometimes people feel serene when:

- They take a long walk in nature
- Meditating in a quiet space
- They look out over a calm lake at sunset
- Enjoying the peace of early morning

I feel serene when...

One recent time I felt serene was...

When that happened I expressed myself by...

Other ways I have expressed serenity are...

When I express serenity it impacts the people around me by...

Next time I feel serene I would like to...

By exploring how I feel and express serenity I have learned about myself...

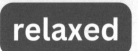

relaxed

being at rest or at ease; free from anxiety

CONNECTED · BELONGING · TRUSTING · SENSITIVE · THANKFUL · LOVING · PEACEFUL · SECURE · SERENE · THOUGHTFUL · INTIMATE · RELAXED · SAFE

Sometimes people feel relaxed when:

- Enjoying a warm bath after a long day
- Lying on a beach listening to the waves
- Reading a book by a cozy fireplace
- They practice deep breathing exercises

I feel relaxed when...

One recent time I felt relaxed was...

When that happened I expressed myself by...

Other ways I have expressed relaxation are...

When I express relaxation it impacts the people around me by...

Next time I feel relaxed I would like to...

By exploring how I feel and express relaxation I have learned about myself...

safe

free from harm or risk; not exposed to danger

CONNECTED
TRUSTING
THANKFUL
SECURE
THOUGHTFUL
INTIMATE
PEACEFUL
BELONGING
SENSITIVE
LOVING
SERENE
RELAXED
SAFE

Sometimes people feel safe when:

- Being in their home where they feel secure
- They have a trusted friend by their side
- Their emotional vulnerabilities are respected
- Their personal boundaries are honored

I feel safe when...

One recent time I felt safe was...   **When that happened I expressed myself by...**

Other ways I have expressed safety are...

When I express safety it impacts the people around me by...   **Next time I feel safe I would like to...**

By exploring how I feel and express safety I have learned about myself...

summary and reflection

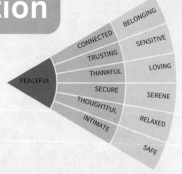

Which feeling was the easiest to write about? Why do you think that is?

Which feeling did you have the most examples for?

Which feeling was the most difficult to write about? Why do you think that is?

Which feeling was the hardest to identify?

What surprised you while journaling about your peaceful feelings?

Did journaling about any of these feelings cause you to feel another feeling?

What have you learned about yourself by journaling about your peaceful feelings?

Sad

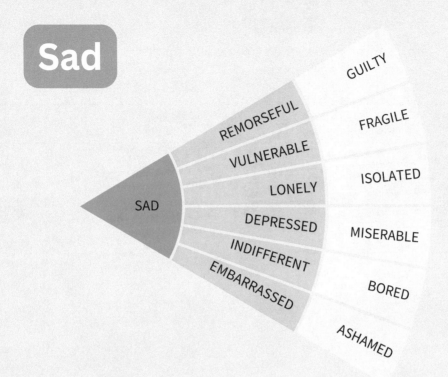

GUILTY
REMORSEFUL
FRAGILE
VULNERABLE
ISOLATED
LONELY
SAD
DEPRESSED
MISERABLE
INDIFFERENT
EMBARRASSED
BORED
ASHAMED

These are some of the feelings in the sad group.
Sometimes when people experience feelings in the sad group
they exhibit the following behaviors:

- Crying or tearing up
- Withdrawing from social activities
- Speaking softly or less frequently
- Showing a lack of interest in usual activities
- Having a decrease in energy or motivation
- Displaying a downcast or forlorn expression
- Having a slower or slumped posture
- Sighing frequently
- Becoming less responsive in conversations
- Exhibiting changes in appetite or sleep patterns

sad

unhappiness, sorrowful or downhearted

Sometimes people feel sad when:

- They go through a breakup or relationship issue
- Suffering from loneliness or isolation
- They face disappointment or failure
- Reflecting on past regrets or missed opportunities

REMORSEFUL
GUILTY
VULNERABLE
FRAGILE
LONELY
ISOLATED
SAD
DEPRESSED
MISERABLE
INDIFFERENT
EMBARRASSED
BORED
ASHAMED

I feel sad when...

One recent time I felt sad was...

When that happened I expressed myself by...

Other ways I have expressed sadness are...

When I express sadness it impacts the people around me by...

Next time I feel sad I would like to...

By exploring how I feel and express sadness I have learned about myself...

remorseful

a sense of guilt for past wrongs

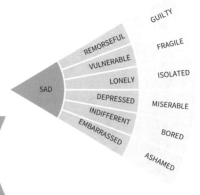

Sometimes people feel remorseful when:

- Realizing they've hurt someone with their actions
- They reflect on a past poor decision
- Apologizing for a mistake that affected a friend
- They lost their temper and said something hurtful

I feel remorseful when...

One recent time I felt remorseful was...

When that happened I expressed myself by...

Other ways I have expressed remorsefulness are...

When I express remorsefulness it impacts the people around me by...

Next time I feel remorseful I would like to...

By exploring how I feel and express remorsefulness I have learned about myself...

vulnerable

exposed to the possibility of being physically or emotionally wounded

Sometimes people feel vulnerable when:

- Sharing a secret and worrying about being judged
- Opening up about their feelings to someone new
- They are recovering from an illness
- Entering a new relationship after being hurt

Emotion wheel labels: SAD, REMORSEFUL, VULNERABLE, LONELY, DEPRESSED, INDIFFERENT, EMBARRASSED, GUILTY, FRAGILE, ISOLATED, MISERABLE, BORED, ASHAMED

I feel vulnerable when...

One recent time I felt vulnerable was...

When that happened I expressed myself by...

Other ways I have expressed vulnerability are...

When I express vulnerability it impacts the people around me by...

Next time I feel vulnerable I would like to...

By exploring how I feel and express vulnerability I have learned about myself...

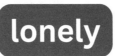

lonely

unhappy due to not being with other people

SAD — REMORSEFUL, VULNERABLE, LONELY, DEPRESSED, INDIFFERENT, EMBARRASSED — GUILTY, FRAGILE, ISOLATED, MISERABLE, BORED, ASHAMED

Sometimes people feel lonely when:

- Spending holidays alone away from family
- They're not invited to a party
- They move to a new city and don't know anyone
- They have difficulty connecting with others

I feel lonely when...

One recent time I felt lonely was...

When that happened I expressed myself by...

Other ways I have expressed loneliness are...

When I express loneliness it impacts the people around me by...

Next time I feel lonely I would like to...

By exploring how I feel and express loneliness I have learned about myself...

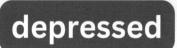

depressed

low in spirits and without hope

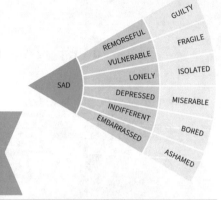

Sometimes people feel depressed when:

- Going through a tough situation in their home life
- A family member, friend, or pet passes away
- Going through a breakup or job loss
- They don't have a support system to lean on

I feel depressed when...

One recent time I felt depressed was...

When that happened I expressed myself by...

Other ways I have expressed depression are...

When I express depression it impacts the people around me by...

Next time I feel depressed I would like to...

By exploring how I feel and express depression I have learned about myself...

indifferent

lack of interest, enthusiasm, or concern

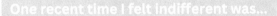

Sometimes people feel indifferent when:

- They are disinterested in participating
- Showing no preference toward different outcomes
- They have a lack of reaction to big news
- Showing no concern for someone else's suffering

I feel indifferent when...

One recent time I felt indifferent was...

When that happened I expressed myself by...

Other ways I have expressed indifference are...

When I express indifference it impacts the people around me by...

Next time I feel indifferent I would like to...

By exploring how I feel and express indifference I have learned about myself...

embarrassed

self-conscious confusion and distress

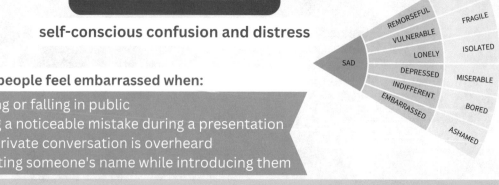

Sometimes people feel embarrassed when:

- Tripping or falling in public
- Making a noticeable mistake during a presentation
- Their private conversation is overheard
- Forgetting someone's name while introducing them

I feel embarrassed when...

One recent time I felt embarrassed

When that happened I expressed myself by...

Other ways I have expressed embarrassment are...

When I express embarrassment it impacts the people around me by...

Next time I feel embarrassed I would like to...

By exploring how I feel and express embarrassment I have learned about myself...

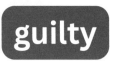

guilty

responsible or regretful for a perceived offense,
real or imaginary

Sometimes people feel guilty when:

GUILTY
REMORSEFUL
VULNERABLE
FRAGILE
LONELY
ISOLATED
DEPRESSED
MISERABLE
INDIFFERENT
EMBARRASSED
BORED
SAD
ASHAMED

- They are dishonest with a friend
- Realizing they forgot their partner's birthday
- They are unable to help a friend in need
- Thinking they're not doing enough for their family

I feel guilty when...

One recent time I felt guilty was...

When that happened I expressed myself by...

Other ways I have expressed guiltiness are...

When I express guiltiness it impacts the people around me by...

Next time I feel guilty I would like to...

By exploring how I feel and express guiltiness I have learned about myself...

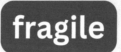

fragile

not strong or sturdy; delicate and vulnerable

GUILTY
REMORSEFUL
FRAGILE
VULNERABLE
ISOLATED
LONELY
SAD
DEPRESSED
MISERABLE
INDIFFERENT
EMBARRASSED
BORED
ASHAMED

Sometimes people feel fragile when:

- They receive a piece of criticism that upsets them
- They are overwhelmed by life's demands
- Recovering from an emotional setback
- Experiencing a sense of vulnerability after an illness

I feel fragile when...

One recent time I felt fragile was...

When that happened I expressed myself by...

Other ways I have expressed fragility are...

When I express fragility it impacts the people around me by...

Next time I feel fragile I would like to...

By exploring how I feel and express fragility I have learned about myself...

isolated

detached from others and unable to connect

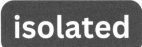

Sometimes people feel isolated when:

- They are in quarantine due to illness
- Being misunderstood by their community
- They live far away from family and friends
- Being excluded from a social group

SAD
REMORSEFUL
VULNERABLE
LONELY
DEPRESSED
INDIFFERENT
EMBARRASSED
GUILTY
FRAGILE
ISOLATED
MISERABLE
BORED
ASHAMED

I feel isolated when...

One recent time I felt isolated was...

When that happened I expressed myself by...

Other ways I have expressed isolation are...

When I express isolation it impacts the people around me by...

Next time I feel isolated I would like to...

By exploring how I feel and express isolation I have learned about myself...

miserable

extremely unhappy or uncomfortable

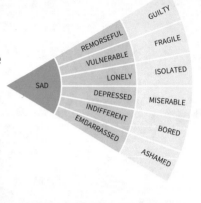

Sometimes people feel miserable when:

- They go through a painful breakup
- Mourning the loss of a loved one
- Suffering through a job they hate
- They are stuck in a toxic living environment

I feel miserable when...

One recent time I felt miserable was...

When that happened I expressed myself by...

Other ways I have expressed miserableness are...

When I express miserableness it impacts the people around me by...

Next time I feel miserable I would like to...

By exploring how I feel and express miserableness I have learned about myself...

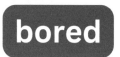

bored

weary and restless through lack of interest

Sometimes people feel bored when:

- They have nothing to do on a weekend
- Performing repetitive tasks with no variation
- They have to wait in a long line with no distractions
- Staying in bed all day with no motivation

GUILTY
REMORSEFUL
FRAGILE
VULNERABLE
ISOLATED
LONELY
DEPRESSED
MISERABLE
INDIFFERENT
EMBARRASSED
BORED
SAD
ASHAMED

I feel bored when...

One recent time I felt bored was...

When that happened I expressed myself by...

Other ways I have expressed boredom are...

When I express boredom it impacts the people around me by...

Next time I feel bored I would like to...

By exploring how I feel and express boredom I have learned about myself...

ashamed

consciousness of guilt, shortcoming, embarrassment or disgrace

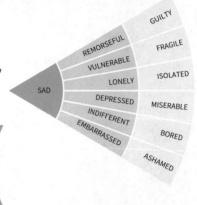

Sometimes people feel ashamed when:

- Being called out for a mistake in front of their peers
- They don't live up to their own moral standards
- A humiliating fact about them is revealed
- Failing at something after boasting about their skill

I feel ashamed when...

One recent time I felt ashamed was...

When that happened I expressed myself by...

Other ways I have expressed shame are...

When I express shame it impacts the people around me by...

Next time I feel ashamed I would like to...

By exploring how I feel and express shame I have learned about myself...

summary and reflection

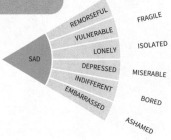

GUILTY
REMORSEFUL
FRAGILE
VULNERABLE
ISOLATED
LONELY
DEPRESSED
MISERABLE
INDIFFERENT
SAD
EMBARRASSED
BORED
ASHAMED

Which feeling was the easiest to write about? Why do you think that is?

Which feeling did you have the most examples for?

Which feeling was the most difficult to write about? Why do you think that is?

Which feeling was the hardest to identify?

What surprised you while journaling about your sad feelings?

Did journaling about any of these feelings cause you to feel another feeling?

What have you learned about yourself by journaling about your sad feelings?

Angry

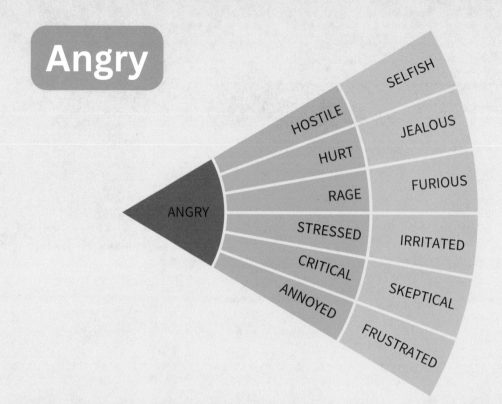

These are some of the feelings in the angry group.
Sometimes when people experience feelings in the angry group they exhibit the following behaviors:

- Frowning or scowling
- Raising their voice or yelling
- Arguing or engaging in verbal disputes
- Showing physical signs of agitation, such as clenched fists
- Becoming withdrawn or silent if anger is turned inward
- Exhibiting sarcasm or cynicism
- Having a sharp or curt tone in conversation
- Stomping, slamming doors, or other forceful movements
- Interrupting or speaking over others
- Fixating on the subject of anger or repeatedly discussing it

angry

strong displeasure, hostility and antagonism

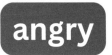

Sometimes people feel angry when:

- They are disrespected or insulted
- Dealing with injustice or unfair treatment
- They experience betrayal or deception
- They receive unfairly harsh criticism

I feel angry when...

One recent time I felt angry was...

When that happened I expressed myself by...

Other ways I have expressed anger are...

When I express anger it impacts the people around me by...

Next time I feel angry I would like to...

By exploring how I feel and express anger I have learned about myself...

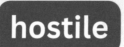

hostile

openly opposed, resisting or aggressive

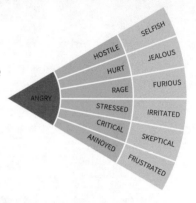

Sometimes people feel hostile when:

- Witnessing the unfair treatment of a friend
- Their ideas are stolen or used without credit
- They are cut off in traffic by an inconsiderate driver
- Being insulted or disrespected by someone

I feel hostile when...

One recent time I felt hostile was...

When that happened I expressed myself by...

Other ways I have expressed hostility are...

When I express hostility it impacts the people around me by...

Next time I feel hostile I would like to...

By exploring how I feel and express hostility I have learned about myself...

hurt

pain, distress or anguish

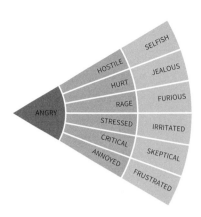

Sometimes people feel hurt when:

- They are betrayed by someone they trusted
- Receiving harsh criticism from a loved one
- Finding out they were excluded from a social event
- They recall a painful memory or experience

I feel hurt when...

One recent time I felt hurt was...

When that happened I expressed myself by...

Other ways I have expressed hurt are...

When I express hurt it impacts the people around me by...

Next time I feel hurt I would like to...

By exploring how I feel and express hurt I have learned about myself...

rage

violent and uncontrolled anger

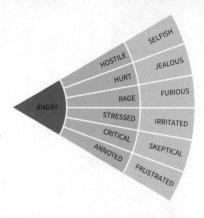

Sometimes people feel rage when:

- Experiencing abuse or profound injustice
- They are the victim of a crime or malicious act
- Their core values are attacked
- Seeing someone they love be hurt or threatened

I feel rage when...

One recent time I felt rage was...

When that happened I expressed myself by...

Other ways I have expressed rage are...

When I express rage it impacts the people around me by...

Next time I feel rage I would like to...

By exploring how I feel and express rage I have learned about myself...

stressed

worried and nervous; bodily or mental tension

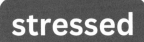

Sometimes people feel stressed when:

- Facing tight deadlines at work or school
- They juggle too many responsibilities at once
- Experiencing ongoing conflict in a relationship
- They cope with a sudden crisis or emergency

I feel stressed when...

One recent time I felt stressed was...

When that happened I expressed myself by...

Other ways I have expressed stress are...

When I express stress it impacts the people around me by...

Next time I feel stressed I would like to...

By exploring how I feel and express stress I have learned about myself...

critical

inclined to find fault or judge with severity

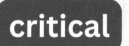

Sometimes people feel critical when:

- They observe someone make repeated mistakes
- Dealing with perceived incompetence at work
- They watch a disappointing movie or show
- Seeing someone disregard advice or warnings

I feel critical when...

One recent time I felt critical was...

When that happened I expressed myself by...

Other ways I have expressed criticalness are...

When I express criticalness it impacts the people around me by...

Next time I feel critical I would like to...

By exploring how I feel and express criticalness I have learned about myself...

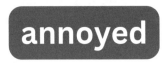

annoyed

angry irritation

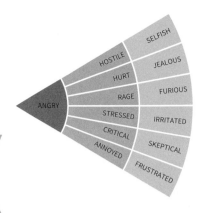

Sometimes people feel annoyed when:

- They endure constant noise from a neighbor's home
- Being repeatedly interrupted while trying to focus
- Dealing with minor but persistent inconveniences
- Someone does not take their requests seriously

I feel annoyed when...

One recent time I felt annoyed was...

When that happened I expressed myself by...

Other ways I have expressed annoyance are...

When I express annoyance it impacts the people around me by...

Next time I feel annoyed I would like to...

By exploring how I feel and express annoyance I have learned about myself...

selfish

concerned excessively or exclusively with oneself

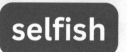

SELFISH
HOSTILE
JEALOUS
HURT
RAGE
FURIOUS
STRESSED
IRRITATED
CRITICAL
ANNOYED
SKEPTICAL
FRUSTRATED
ANGRY

Sometimes people feel selfish when:

- They put their own needs above everyone else's
- Talking about themselves constantly
- They ignore community rules for personal gain
- They take credit for someone else's work

I feel selfish when...

One recent time I felt selfish was...

When that happened I expressed myself by...

Other ways I have expressed selfishness are...

When I express selfishness it impacts the people around me by...

Next time I feel selfish I would like to...

By exploring how I feel and express selfishness I have learned about myself...

jealous

hostile and intolerant; resentful and bitter

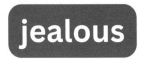

Sometimes people feel jealous when:

- Their partner seems interested in another person
- A peer receives widespread praise
- Their partner receives attention from someone else
- Struggling with a goal that a peer easily achieves

I feel jealous when...

One recent time I felt jealous was...

When that happened I expressed myself by...

Other ways I have expressed jealousy are...

When I express jealousy it impacts the people around me by...

Next time I feel jealous I would like to...

By exploring how I feel and express jealousy I have learned about myself...

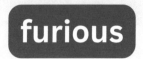

furious

extremely angry

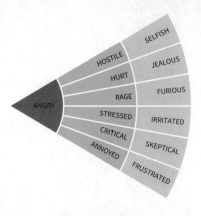

Sometimes people feel furious when:

- They discover deceit or lies from a trusted person
- Their property is deliberately damaged
- Facing repeated injustice or discrimination
- They watch someone put others at risk

I feel furious when...

One recent time I felt furious was...

When that happened I expressed myself by...

Other ways I have expressed furiousness are...

When I express furiousness it impacts the people around me by...

Next time I feel furious I would like to...

By exploring how I feel and express furiousness I have learned about myself...

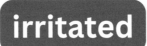

irritated

displeased or bothered by something or someone

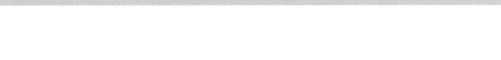

Sometimes people feel irritated when:

- They deal with seasonal allergies
- Having to correct the same mistake multiple times
- They are subjected to unwanted advice
- Encountering delays in a service they're paying for

I feel irritated when...

One recent time I felt irritated was...

When that happened I expressed myself by...

Other ways I have expressed irritation are...

When I express irritation it impacts the people around me by...

Next time I feel irritated I would like to...

By exploring how I feel and express irritation I have learned about myself...

skeptical

doubting that something is true or useful

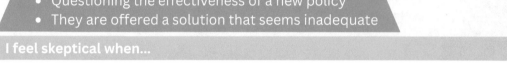

Sometimes people feel skeptical when:

- They hear claims that seem too good to be true
- They doubt the sincerity of someone's apology
- Questioning the effectiveness of a new policy
- They are offered a solution that seems inadequate

I feel skeptical when...

One recent time I felt skeptical was...

When that happened I expressed myself by...

Other ways I have expressed skepticism are...

When I express skepticism it impacts the people around me by...

Next time I feel skeptical I would like to...

By exploring how I feel and express skepticism I have learned about myself...

frustrated

annoyed, disappointed and discouraged

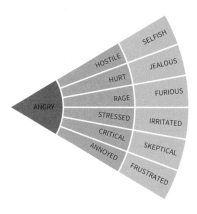

Sometimes people feel frustrated when:

- They have unresolved problems or unfulfilled needs
- Encountering repeated obstacles
- They are unable to solve a challenging issue at work
- Experiencing a lack of cooperation from a team

I feel frustrated when...

One recent time I felt frustrated was...   **When that happened I expressed myself by...**

Other ways I have expressed frustration are...

When I express frustration it impacts the people around me by...   **Next time I feel frustrated I would like to...**

By exploring how I feel and express frustration I have learned about myself...

summary and reflection

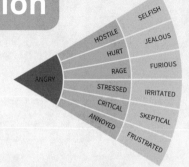

HOSTILE
SELFISH
HURT
JEALOUS
RAGE
FURIOUS
ANGRY
STRESSED
IRRITATED
CRITICAL
SKEPTICAL
ANNOYED
FRUSTRATED

Which feeling was the easiest to write about? Why do you think that is?

Which feeling did you have the most examples for?

Which feeling was the most difficult to write about? Why do you think that is?

Which feeling was the hardest to identify?

What surprised you while journaling about your angry feelings?

Did journaling about any of these feelings cause you to feel another feeling?

What have you learned about yourself by journaling about your angry feelings?

Scared

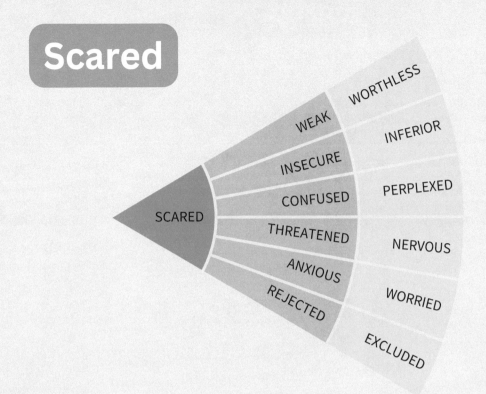

These are some of the feelings in the scared group. Sometimes when people experience feelings in the scared group they exhibit the following behaviors:

- Exhibiting nervous habits like nail-biting or fidgeting
- Showing hesitancy or reluctance to engage in certain activities
- Having a startled or jumpy reaction to unexpected events
- Avoiding situations or places that evoke fear
- Seeking reassurance from others
- Displaying increased vigilance or alertness
- Having difficulty concentrating on tasks
- Experiencing physical symptoms such as sweating or trembling
- Expressing worry or voicing concerns frequently
- Looking for escape routes or exit strategies

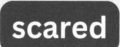

scared

frightened, worried, afraid; in fear

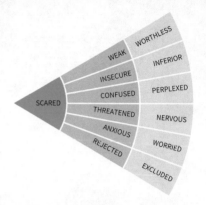

Sometimes people feel scared when:

- Facing a threatening or unknown situation
- They anticipate a negative outcome
- Experiencing instability or insecurity
- They encounter a phobia or fear trigger

I feel scared when...

One recent time I felt scared was...

When that happened I expressed myself by...

Other ways I have expressed scaredness are...

When I express scaredness it impacts the people around me by...

Next time I feel scared I would like to...

By exploring how I feel and express scaredness I have learned about myself...

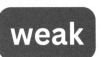

weak

**not strong in character; unable to make decisions
or to persuade or lead other people**

Sometimes people feel weak when:

- They are unable to defend themself
- Struggling to walk after a strenuous workout
- Experiencing helplessness during an anxiety attack
- They are exhausted after a long period of stress

WEAK
WORTHLESS
INFERIOR
INSECURE
CONFUSED
PERPLEXED
SCARED
THREATENED
NERVOUS
ANXIOUS
WORRIED
REJECTED
EXCLUDED

I feel weak when...

One recent time I felt weak was...

When that happened I expressed myself by...

Other ways I have expressed weakness are...

When I express weakness it impacts the people around me by...

Next time I feel weak I would like to...

By exploring how I feel and express weakness I have learned about myself...

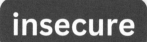

insecure

lacking confidence and doubting one's own abilities

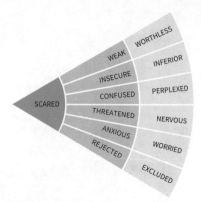

Sometimes people feel insecure when:

- Doubting their abilities before a presentation
- Not believing they measure up to their peers
- Worrying about the stability of their relationships
- Experiencing self-doubt while scrolling social media

I feel insecure when...

One recent time I felt insecure was...

When that happened I expressed myself by...

Other ways I have expressed insecurity are...

When I express insecurity it impacts the people around me by...

Next time I feel insecure I would like to...

By exploring how I feel and express insecurity I have learned about myself...

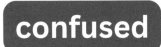

confused

unable to think clearly or to understand something

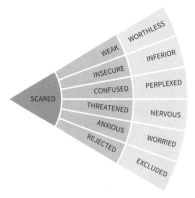

Sometimes people feel confused when:

- They receive contradictory advice
- Trying to understand a complex subject
- They misunderstand directions and get lost
- Witnessing a friend's contradictory behavior

I feel confused when...

One recent time I felt confused was...

When that happened I expressed myself by...

Other ways I have expressed confusion are...

When I express confusion it impacts the people around me by...

Next time I feel confused I would like to...

By exploring how I feel and express confusion I have learned about myself...

threatened

in danger or suspecting that something bad might happen

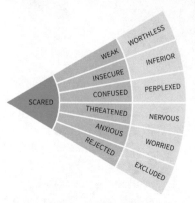

Sometimes people feel threatened when:

- They walk alone at night in an unsafe area
- Being bullied or intimidated by someone
- They face the possibility of losing their job
- Observing escalating hostility in their environment

I feel threatened when...

One recent time I felt threatened was...

When that happened I expressed myself by...

Other ways I have expressed threat are...

When I express threat it impacts the people around me by...

Next time I feel threatened I would like to...

By exploring how I feel and express threat I have learned about myself...

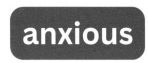

anxious

worried and nervous

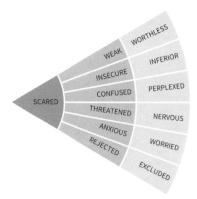

Sometimes people feel anxious when:

- They wait for the results of a test
- Preparing to speak in front of a large audience
- They approach a deadline for a project
- Preparing to meet their partner's parents

I feel anxious when...

One recent time I felt anxious was...

When that happened I expressed myself by...

Other ways I have expressed anxiety are...

When I express anxiety it impacts the people around me by...

Next time I feel anxious I would like to...

By exploring how I feel and express anxiety I have learned about myself...

rejected

not receiving love, attention or acceptance

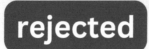

Sometimes people feel rejected when:

- They don't get a job after an interview goes well
- They are turned down by someone they asked out
- Having an idea dismissed without consideration
- They are left out of a social event

I feel rejected when...

One recent time I felt rejected was...

When that happened I expressed myself by...

Other ways I have expressed rejection are...

When I express rejection it impacts the people around me by...

Next time I feel rejected I would like to...

By exploring how I feel and express rejection I have learned about myself...

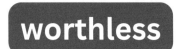

worthless

not important or not useful

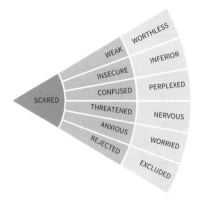

Sometimes people feel worthless when:

- They are criticized harshly and repeatedly
- Comparing themself unfavorably to peers
- They believe their contributions are not valued
- Suffering from a depressive episode

I feel worthless when...

One recent time I felt worthless was...

When that happened I expressed myself by...

Other ways I have expressed worthlessness are...

When I express worthlessness it impacts the people around me by...

Next time I feel worthless I would like to...

By exploring how I feel and express worthlessness I have learned about myself...

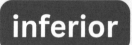

inferior

not as good as someone or something else

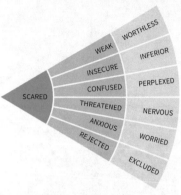

Sometimes people feel inferior when:

- Being treated less than because of their background
- Inadequately comparing themself to someone else
- They receive a poor performance evaluation
- Being excluded because they don't appear to fit in

I feel inferior when...

One recent time I felt inferior was...

When that happened I expressed myself by...

Other ways I have expressed inferiority are...

When I express inferiority it impacts the people around me by...

Next time I feel inferior I would like to...

By exploring how I feel and express inferiority I have learned about myself...

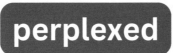

perplexed

confused or filled with uncertainty

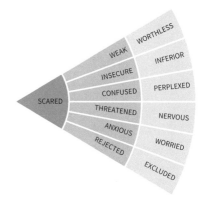

Sometimes people feel perplexed when:

- Something is difficult to understand or solve
- They encounter an unexpected situation
- Failing to understand someone's actions
- They are presented with confusing instructions

I feel perplexed when...

One recent time I felt perplexed was...   **When that happened I expressed myself by...**

Other ways I have expressed perplexity are...

When I express perplexity it impacts the people around me by...   **Next time I feel perplexed I would like to...**

By exploring how I feel and express perplexity I have learned about myself...

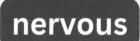

nervous

worried or slightly frightened; timid or apprehensive

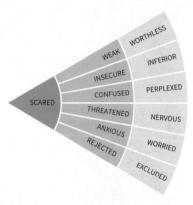

Sometimes people feel nervous when:

- Anticipating a difficult conversation with a friend
- Waiting to hear if they made it through an audition
- They have to navigate a challenging driving route
- Preparing to take an important exam or test

I feel nervous when...

One recent time I felt nervous was...

When that happened I expressed myself by...

Other ways I have expressed nervousness are...

When I express nervousness it impacts the people around me by...

Next time I feel nervous I would like to...

By exploring how I feel and express nervousness I have learned about myself...

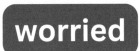

worried

anxious or troubled about actual or potential problems

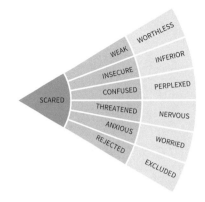

Sometimes people feel worried when:

- Concerned about the well-being of a loved one
- Fearing the outcome of political or social unrest
- They are thinking about environmental issues
- Concerned about making a good impression

I feel worried when...

One recent time I felt worried was...

When that happened I expressed myself by...

Other ways I have expressed worry are...

When I express worry it impacts the people around me by...

Next time I feel worried I would like to...

By exploring how I feel and express worry I have learned about myself...

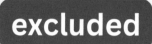

excluded

intentionally not included in something

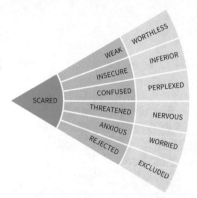

Sometimes people feel excluded when:

- Being the only team member not included in a lunch
- Not being considered for a project or position
- They are consistently ignored in conversations
- They find out they weren't invited to a friend's party

I feel excluded when...

One recent time I felt excluded was...

When that happened I expressed myself by...

Other ways I have expressed exclusion are...

When I express exclusion it impacts the people around me by...

Next time I feel excluded I would like to...

By exploring how I feel and express exclusion I have learned about myself...

summary and reflection

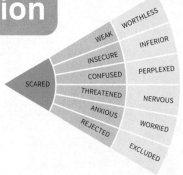

Which feeling was the easiest to write about? Why do you think that is?

Which feeling did you have the most examples for?

Which feeling was the most difficult to write about? Why do you think that is?

Which feeling was the hardest to identify?

What surprised you while journaling about your scared feelings?

Did journaling about any of these feelings cause you to feel another feeling?

What have you learned about yourself by journaling about your scared feelings?

FEELINGS TOOL KIT

GUILTY

FRAGILE

SH

HOSTILE

HURT

RAGE

STRESSED

SK

FRUSTRA

CRITICAL

ANNOYED

WORTHLES

INFERIOR

REMORSE

WEAK

PERPLEXE

ATED

VULNERABLE

INSECURE

NE

LONELY

CONFUSED

E

DEPRESSED

THREATENED

INDIFFERENT

ANXIOUS

EMBARRASSED

REJECTED

E

CONNECTED

PEACEFUL

HAPPY

OPTIMISTIC

TRUSTING

EXCITED

E

THANKFUL

POWERFUL

PLAYFUL

SECURE

CONTENT

AR

THOUGHTFUL

ACCEPTED

INTIMATE

EMPOWERED

APPRECIATED

COURAGEOUS

INTERESTED

JOYFU

ENE

FAITHFUL

STRONG

PROUD

RELAXED

VALUED

SAFE

CURIOUS

FOCUSED

SUCCESSFUL

CONFIDENT

LOYAL

RESPECTED

CREATIVE

The Feelings Wheel

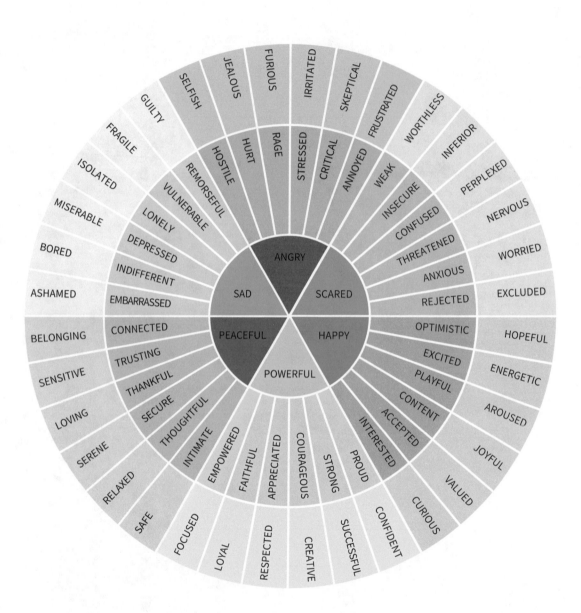

Feelings Iceberg

Just like an iceberg, many of the feelings connected to a core feeling are hidden beneath the surface. Once you identify a core feeling, try to explore it a little deeper and see if you can discover the more specific feelings you are experiencing.

HAPPY

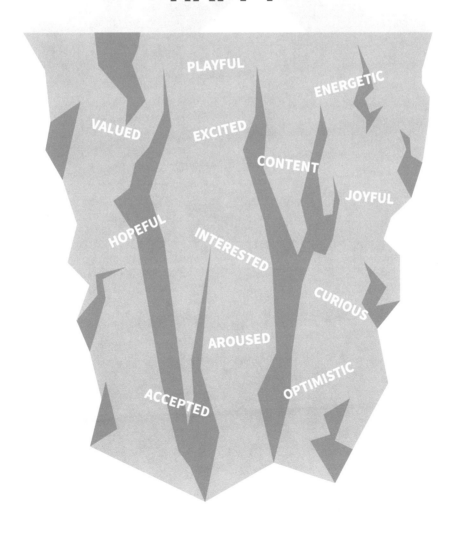

Feelings Iceberg

Just like an iceberg, many of the feelings connected to a core feeling are hidden beneath the surface. Once you identify a core feeling, try to explore it a little deeper and see if you can discover the more specific feelings you are experiencing.

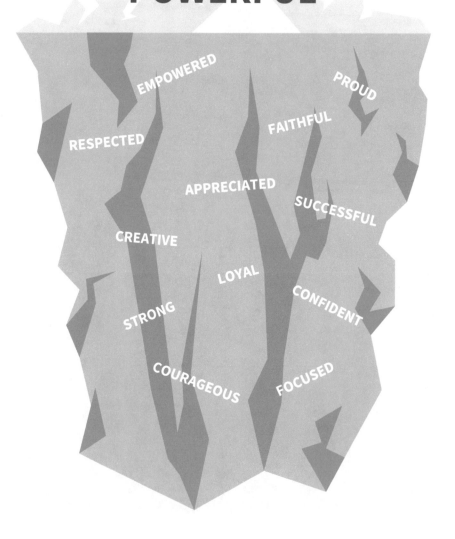

POWERFUL

EMPOWERED

PROUD

FAITHFUL

RESPECTED

APPRECIATED

SUCCESSFUL

CREATIVE

LOYAL

STRONG

CONFIDENT

COURAGEOUS

FOCUSED

Feelings Iceberg

Just like an iceberg, many of the feelings connected to a core feeling are hidden beneath the surface. Once you identify a core feeling, try to explore it a little deeper and see if you can discover the more specific feelings you are experiencing.

PEACEFUL

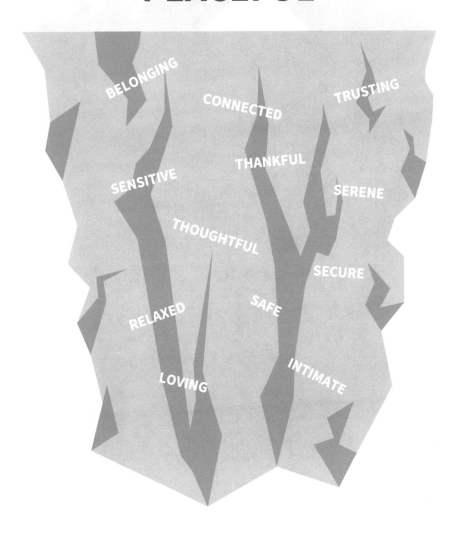

Feelings Iceberg

Just like an iceberg, many of the feelings connected to a core feeling are hidden beneath the surface. Once you identify a core feeling, try to explore it a little deeper and see if you can discover the more specific feelings you are experiencing.

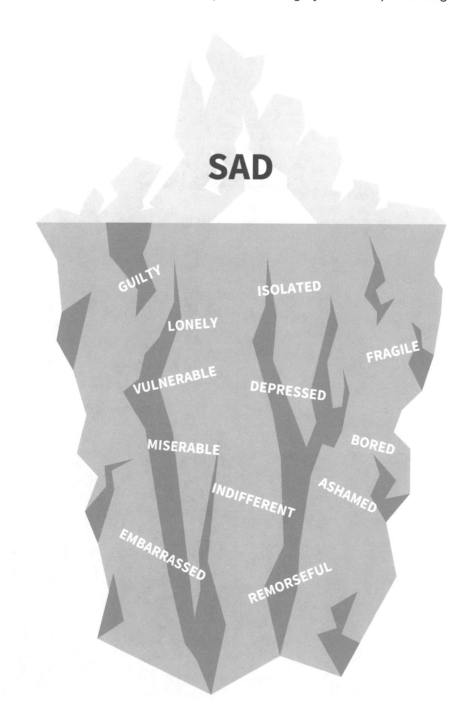

SAD

GUILTY

ISOLATED

LONELY

FRAGILE

VULNERABLE

DEPRESSED

MISERABLE

BORED

INDIFFERENT

ASHAMED

EMBARRASSED

REMORSEFUL

Feelings Iceberg

Just like an iceberg, many of the feelings connected to a core feeling are hidden beneath the surface. Once you identify a core feeling, try to explore it a little deeper and see if you can discover the more specific feelings you are experiencing.

ANGRY

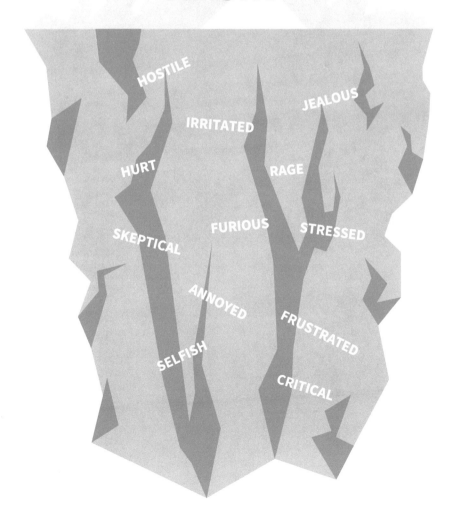

Feelings Iceberg

Just like an iceberg, many of the feelings connected to a core feeling are hidden beneath the surface. Once you identify a core feeling, try to explore it a little deeper and see if you can discover the more specific feelings you are experiencing.

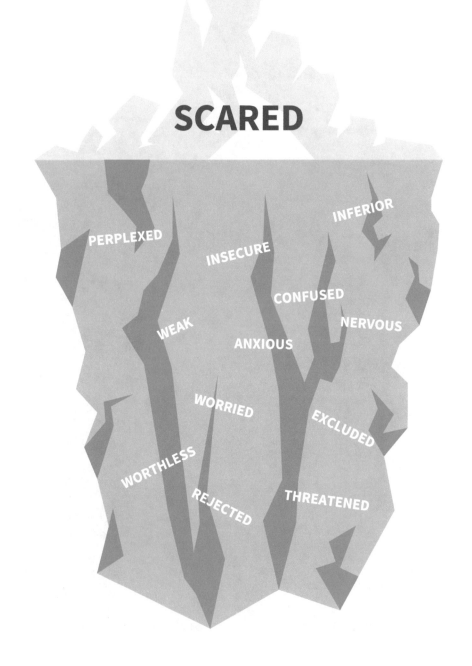

SCARED

PERPLEXED

INFERIOR

INSECURE

CONFUSED

WEAK

NERVOUS

ANXIOUS

WORRIED

EXCLUDED

WORTHLESS

REJECTED

THREATENED

Gauging Complex Feelings

Use the thermometers to gauge your feelings in each of the core areas. Once you've identified which core feeling you're experiencing the strongest, look at the Feelings Wheel or Feelings Iceberg to see if you can identify any specific feelings hiding below the surface. Repeat this for each core area in which you are experiencing feelings.

10	10	10	10	10	10
9	9	9	9	9	9
8	8	8	8	8	8
7	7	7	7	7	7
6	6	6	6	6	6
5	5	5	5	5	5
4	4	4	4	4	4
3	3	3	3	3	3
2	2	2	2	2	2
1	1	1	1	1	1

| SAD | ANGRY | SCARED | HAPPY | PEACEFUL | POWERFUL |

Feelings Body Scan

Take a few deep breaths and close your eyes (if you feel safe enough to do so).
Become aware of your 5 senses (sight, sound, smell, taste, touch/feel).
Identify where you feel the feeling in your body and notice any sensations that arise.

Begin at the top of your head and end at the bottom of your toes.

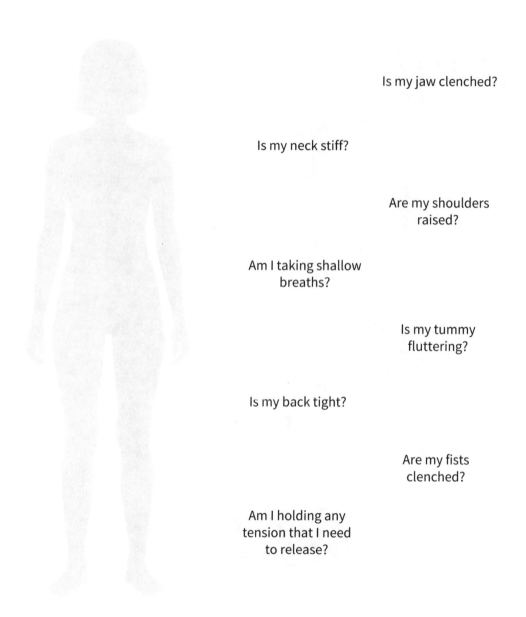

Is my jaw clenched?

Is my neck stiff?

Are my shoulders raised?

Am I taking shallow breaths?

Is my tummy fluttering?

Is my back tight?

Are my fists clenched?

Am I holding any tension that I need to release?

Stretch, move, massage, shake or breathe into the areas of your body that are holding tension.

Feeling Feelings

As you experience a feeling, try to locate where you feel it in your body.
Use the Feelings Body Scan as a guide.

Where do you feel the feeling in your body?

What do you think your body is telling you?

How can you care for yourself as you process this feeling?

Validating Feelings

All feelings are okay to have and every feeling you experience is valid. There is no such thing as a "good" or "bad" feeling. As you are learning about the feelings you experience, be sure to validate those feelings and allow yourself space to feel them as they come and go.

Use this tool to practice validating your feelings.

I feel _____(insert feeling).

It's okay that I feel _____(insert feeling).

I'm allowed to feel _____(insert feeling).

I give myself permission to feel _____(insert feeling).

I feel _____(insert feeling).

It's okay that I feel _____(insert feeling).

I'm allowed to feel _____(insert feeling).

I give myself permission to feel _____(insert feeling).

Processing Feelings

1. AWARENESS

The first step is becoming aware that you're experiencing a feeling.

2. IDENTIFICATION

The next step is identifying what the feeling is and naming it. You can use the Feelings Wheel to help with this.

3. ATTRIBUTION

Then you can start to make sense of what caused the feeling. You can use the Thoughts/Feelings/Behaviors Triangle to help chart it out.

4. ACCEPTANCE

Check-in with yourself and notice any related physical sensations in your body. Accept the feeling as valid, allow yourself to experience it.

5. ACTION

Take a few deep breaths and then decide what you will do. Choose how you will use or cope with the feeling. Choose how you will express it.

Thoughts / Feelings / Behaviors Triangle

This is a tool that may help you start to make sense of what causes your feelings.
Please seek the guidance of a licensed mental health professional if you would like help using this tool.

Thoughts create feelings

Behaviors reinforce thoughts

Feelings create behaviors

Cognitive Reframing

This is a technique that may help you modify your Thoughts/Feelings/Behaviors pattern.
Please seek the guidance of a licensed mental health professional if you would like help using this technique.

SITUATION
a short description of what happened - only the facts

> *Example: When I walked into the room, I smiled and waved at my friend. She did not wave back or smile.*

	MY ACTUAL THOUGHT	**ALTERNATE THOUGHT**
THOUGHTS interpret the situation using your thoughts (note that interpretations are not always accurate - there are many ways to think about the same situation)	*Example: She is clearly mad at me. And embarrassed that we are friends. She doesn't want anyone to know that she is friends with me.*	*Example: She is not responding in a way that is normal for her. I wonder if she is going through something right now.*
FEELINGS identify the feelings you experience as a result of your actual thought - and the ones you may have with the alternate thought (you can use the Feelings Wheel to help with this)	*Example: Embarrassed, insecure, rejected, excluded.*	*Example: Curious, secure, thoughtful, trusting.*
BEHAVIOR decide how you will use, cope with or express your feelings - do this for the feelings connected to your actual thought and your alternate thought	*Example: Ignore her texts and calls. Avoid places she usually goes so I don't feel embarrassed again.*	*Example: Call her later to check on her. Invite her to lunch so she knows that she's not alone, even if she's going through something she doesn't want to talk about.*

Coping With Feelings

Here are 50 actions that may help you cope with challenging feelings:

- go for a walk
- call a friend
- spend time in nature
- turn off your phone
- drink water
- write a gratitude list
- do a puzzle
- go for a drive
- exercise or move your body
- cuddle with your pet
- give yourself a pep talk
- write some affirmations
- dance to your favorite songs
- do a mindfulness exercise
- take a mental health day
- find a support group
- take a break from social media
- do something to help someone else
- ask for help from a loved one
- look through old photos
- sew, crochet or knit
- set boundaries
- have a spa day at home
- watch a movie or show you love
- reflect on your spiritual beliefs
- spend 10 minutes meditating
- use a weighted blanket
- make a vision board
- spend time with a loved one
- celebrate yourself
- volunteer in your community
- learn a new skill or hobby
- cook or bake using a new recipe
- squeeze a stress ball
- plan something fun to look forward to
- play a board game or video game
- focus on what is in your control
- light candles
- set a small goal
- diffuse essential oils
- clean or organize your space
- buy some new plants
- make a playlist of songs you love
- read a book
- try a new food or cuisine
- listen to some sounds from nature
- create a routine or schedule
- walk in the grass barefoot
- play a sport
- name 5 things you love about yourself

PRACTICE PAGES

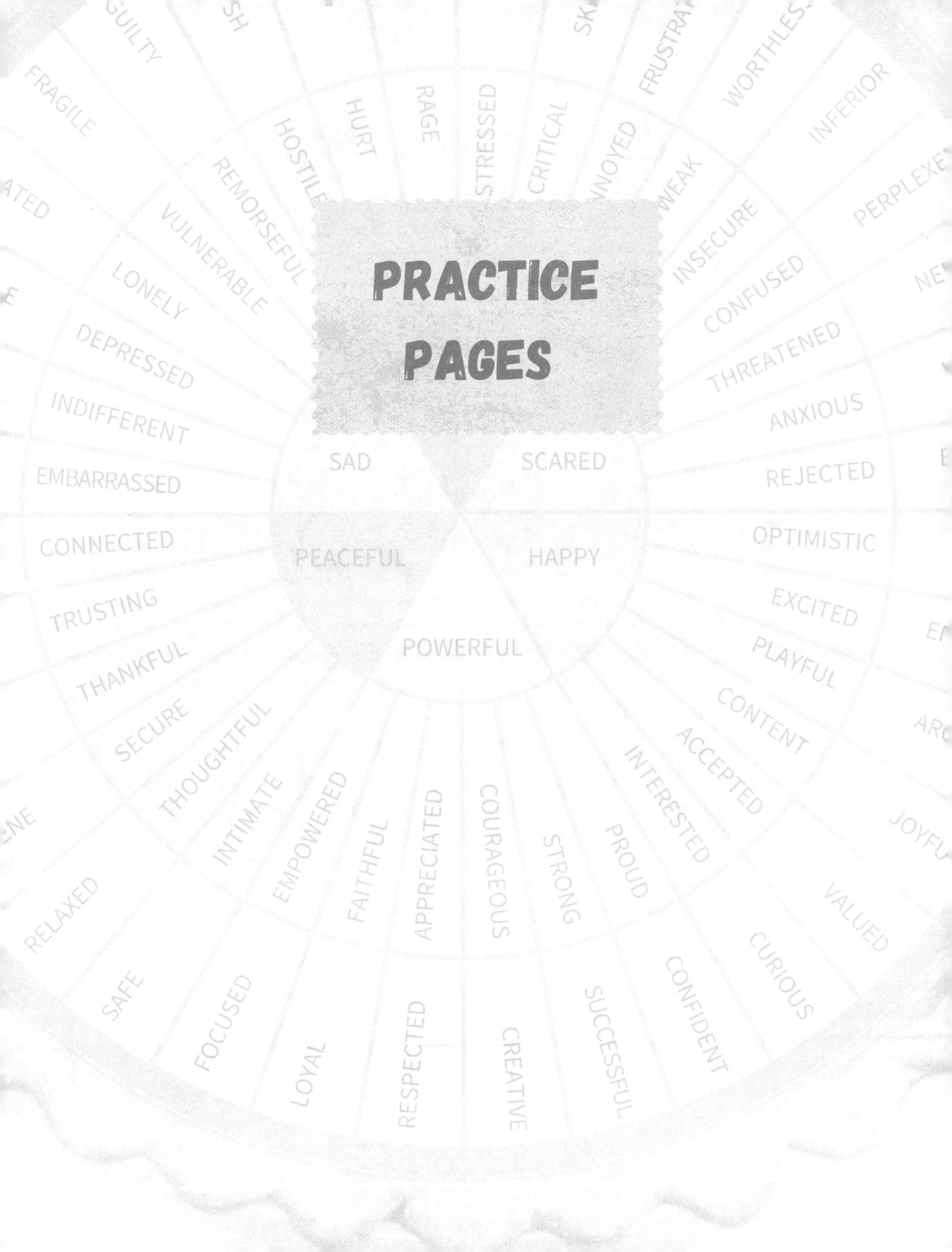

Feelings Pie Challenge

There are so many more feelings than what we covered on the Feelings Wheel in this journal. How many more feelings can you identify? Write them in the blank spaces here.

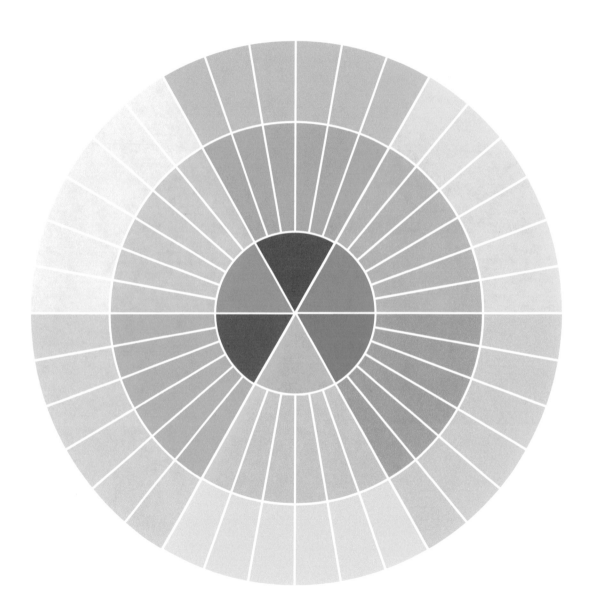

Gauging Complex Feelings

Use the thermometers to gauge your feelings in each of the core areas. Once you've identified which core feeling you're experiencing the strongest, look at the Feelings Wheel or Feelings Iceberg to see if you can identify any specific feelings hiding below the surface. Repeat this for each core area in which you are experiencing feelings.

SAD	ANGRY	SCARED	HAPPY	PEACEFUL	POWERFUL
10	10	10	10	10	10
9	9	9	9	9	9
8	8	8	8	8	8
7	7	7	7	7	7
6	6	6	6	6	6
5	5	5	5	5	5
4	4	4	4	4	4
3	3	3	3	3	3
2	2	2	2	2	2
1	1	1	1	1	1

Gauging Complex Feelings

Use the thermometers to gauge your feelings in each of the core areas. Once you've identified which core feeling you're experiencing the strongest, look at the Feelings Wheel or Feelings Iceberg to see if you can identify any specific feelings hiding below the surface. Repeat this for each core area in which you are experiencing feelings.

10	10	10	10	10	10
9	9	9	9	9	9
8	8	8	8	8	8
7	7	7	7	7	7
6	6	6	6	6	6
5	5	5	5	5	5
4	4	4	4	4	4
3	3	3	3	3	3
2	2	2	2	2	2
1	1	1	1	1	1

| SAD | ANGRY | SCARED | HAPPY | PEACEFUL | POWERFUL |

Gauging Complex Feelings

Use the thermometers to gauge your feelings in each of the core areas. Once you've identified which core feeling you're experiencing the strongest, look at the Feelings Wheel or Feelings Iceberg to see if you can identify any specific feelings hiding below the surface. Repeat this for each core area in which you are experiencing feelings.

SAD	ANGRY	SCARED	HAPPY	PEACEFUL	POWERFUL

Gauging Complex Feelings

Use the thermometers to gauge your feelings in each of the core areas. Once you've identified which core feeling you're experiencing the strongest, look at the Feelings Wheel or Feelings Iceberg to see if you can identify any specific feelings hiding below the surface. Repeat this for each core area in which you are experiencing feelings.

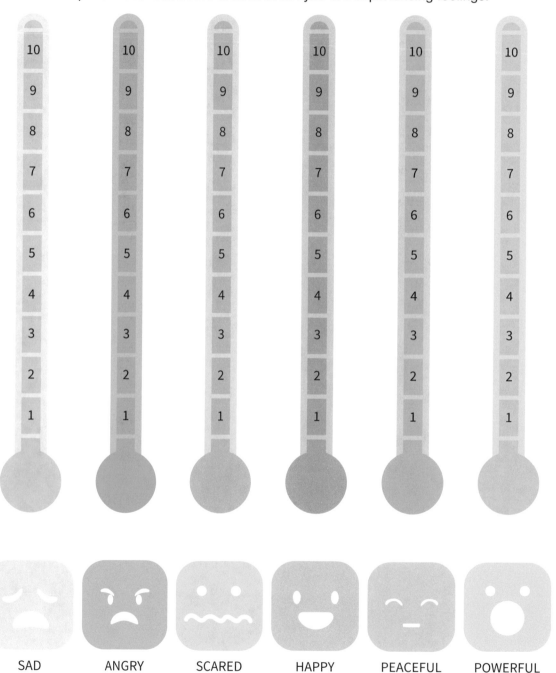

Gauging Complex Feelings

Use the thermometers to gauge your feelings in each of the core areas. Once you've identified which core feeling you're experiencing the strongest, look at the Feelings Wheel or Feelings Iceberg to see if you can identify any specific feelings hiding below the surface. Repeat this for each core area in which you are experiencing feelings.

SAD	ANGRY	SCARED	HAPPY	PEACEFUL	POWERFUL
10	10	10	10	10	10
9	9	9	9	9	9
8	8	8	8	8	8
7	7	7	7	7	7
6	6	6	6	6	6
5	5	5	5	5	5
4	4	4	4	4	4
3	3	3	3	3	3
2	2	2	2	2	2
1	1	1	1	1	1

Feeling My Feelings

As you experience a feeling, try to locate where you feel it in your body.
Use the Feelings Body Scan as a guide.

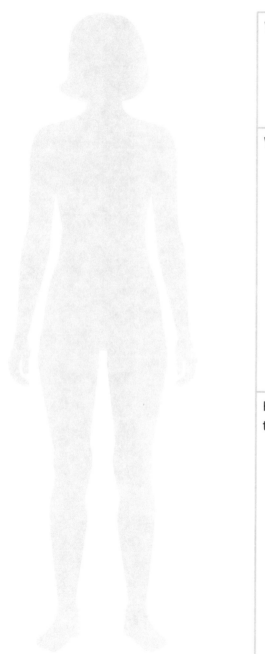

Where do you feel the feeling in your body?

What do you think your body is telling you?

How can you care for yourself as you process this feeling?

Feeling My Feelings

As you experience a feeling, try to locate where you feel it in your body.
Use the Feelings Body Scan as a guide.

Where do you feel the feeling in your body?

What do you think your body is telling you?

How can you care for yourself as you process this feeling?

Feeling My Feelings

As you experience a feeling, try to locate where you feel it in your body.
Use the Feelings Body Scan as a guide.

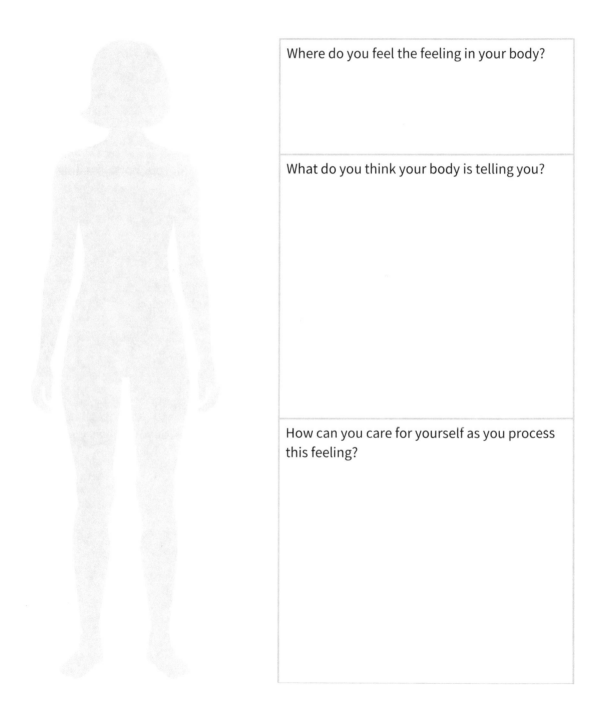

Where do you feel the feeling in your body?

What do you think your body is telling you?

How can you care for yourself as you process this feeling?

Feeling My Feelings

As you experience a feeling, try to locate where you feel it in your body.
Use the Feelings Body Scan as a guide.

Where do you feel the feeling in your body?

What do you think your body is telling you?

How can you care for yourself as you process this feeling?

Feeling My Feelings

As you experience a feeling, try to locate where you feel it in your body.
Use the Feelings Body Scan as a guide.

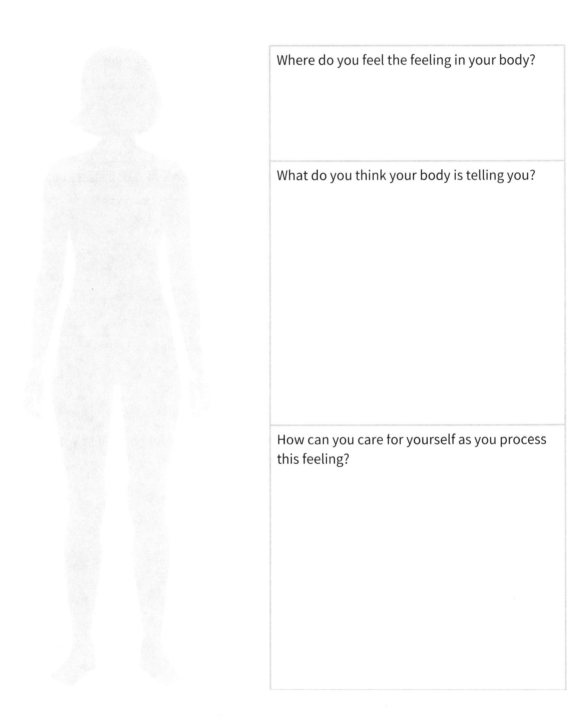

Where do you feel the feeling in your body?

What do you think your body is telling you?

How can you care for yourself as you process this feeling?

Validating Feelings

All feelings are okay to have and every feeling you experience is valid. There is no such thing as a "good" or "bad" feeling. As you are learning about the feelings you experience, be sure to validate those feelings and allow yourself space to feel them as they come and go.

Use this tool to practice validating your feelings.

I feel _____(insert feeling).

It's okay that I feel _____(insert feeling).

I'm allowed to feel _____(insert feeling).

I give myself permission to feel _____(insert feeling).

I feel _____(insert feeling).

It's okay that I feel _____(insert feeling).

I'm allowed to feel _____(insert feeling).

I give myself permission to feel _____(insert feeling).

Validating Feelings

All feelings are okay to have and every feeling you experience is valid. There is no such thing as a "good" or "bad" feeling. As you are learning about the feelings you experience, be sure to validate those feelings and allow yourself space to feel them as they come and go.

Use this tool to practice validating your feelings.

I feel _____(insert feeling).

It's okay that I feel _____(insert feeling).

I'm allowed to feel _____(insert feeling).

I give myself permission to feel _____(insert feeling).

I feel _____(insert feeling).

It's okay that I feel _____(insert feeling).

I'm allowed to feel _____(insert feeling).

I give myself permission to feel _____(insert feeling).

Validating Feelings

All feelings are okay to have and every feeling you experience is valid. There is no such thing as a "good" or "bad" feeling. As you are learning about the feelings you experience, be sure to validate those feelings and allow yourself space to feel them as they come and go.

Use this tool to practice validating your feelings.

I feel _____(*insert feeling*).

It's okay that I feel _____(*insert feeling*).

I'm allowed to feel _____(*insert feeling*).

I give myself permission to feel _____(*insert feeling*).

I feel _____(*insert feeling*).

It's okay that I feel _____(*insert feeling*).

I'm allowed to feel _____(*insert feeling*).

I give myself permission to feel _____(*insert feeling*).

Validating Feelings

All feelings are okay to have and every feeling you experience is valid. There is no such thing as a "good" or "bad" feeling. As you are learning about the feelings you experience, be sure to validate those feelings and allow yourself space to feel them as they come and go.

Use this tool to practice validating your feelings.

I feel _____(*insert feeling*).

It's okay that I feel _____(*insert feeling*).

I'm allowed to feel _____(*insert feeling*).

I give myself permission to feel _____(*insert feeling*).

I feel _____(*insert feeling*).

It's okay that I feel _____(*insert feeling*).

I'm allowed to feel _____(*insert feeling*).

I give myself permission to feel _____(*insert feeling*).

Validating Feelings

All feelings are okay to have and every feeling you experience is valid. There is no such thing as a "good" or "bad" feeling. As you are learning about the feelings you experience, be sure to validate those feelings and allow yourself space to feel them as they come and go.

Use this tool to practice validating your feelings.

I feel _____(*insert feeling*).

It's okay that I feel _____(*insert feeling*).

I'm allowed to feel _____(*insert feeling*).

I give myself permission to feel _____(*insert feeling*).

I feel _____(*insert feeling*).

It's okay that I feel _____(*insert feeling*).

I'm allowed to feel _____(*insert feeling*).

I give myself permission to feel _____(*insert feeling*).

Thoughts / Feelings / Behaviors Triangle

This is a tool that may help you start to make sense of what causes your feelings.
*Please seek the guidance of a licensed mental health professional if you would
like help using this tool.*

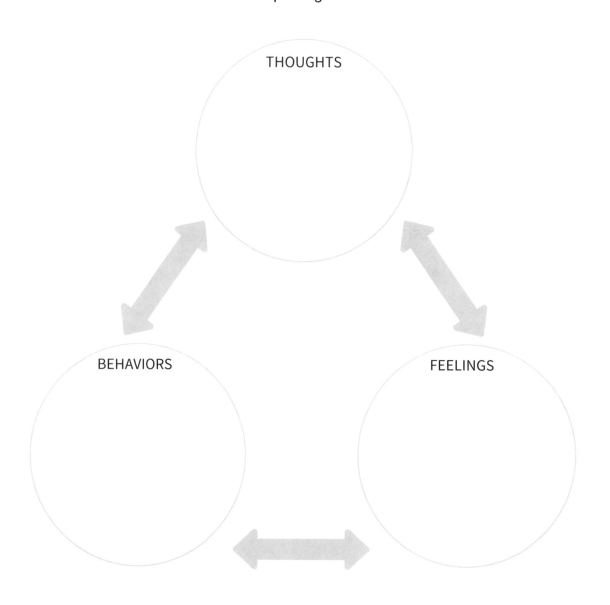

THOUGHTS

BEHAVIORS

FEELINGS

Thoughts / Feelings / Behaviors Triangle

This is a tool that may help you start to make sense of what causes your feelings.
Please seek the guidance of a licensed mental health professional if you would like help using this tool.

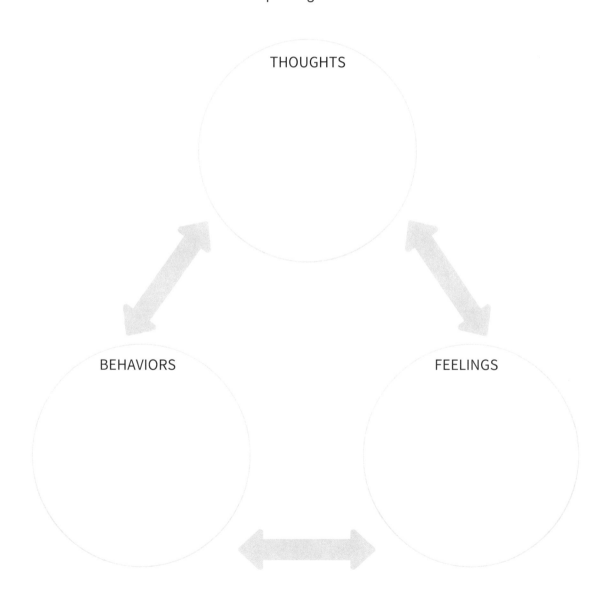

Thoughts / Feelings / Behaviors Triangle

This is a tool that may help you start to make sense of what causes your feelings. *Please seek the guidance of a licensed mental health professional if you would like help using this tool.*

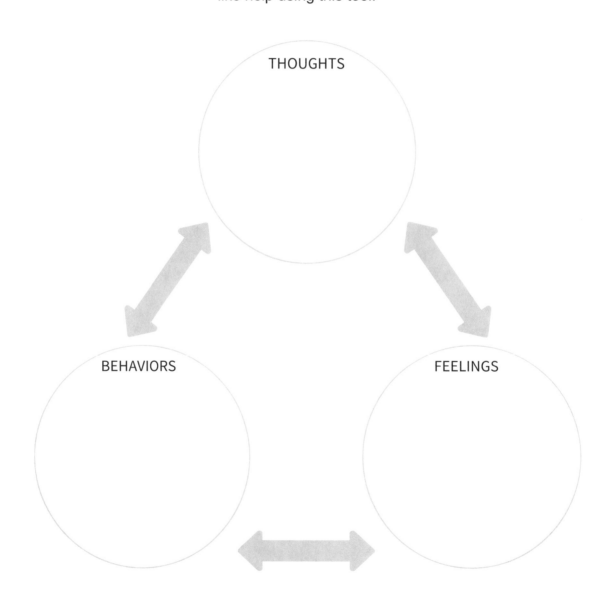

THOUGHTS

BEHAVIORS

FEELINGS

Thoughts / Feelings / Behaviors Triangle

This is a tool that may help you start to make sense of what causes your feelings.
Please seek the guidance of a licensed mental health professional if you would like help using this tool.

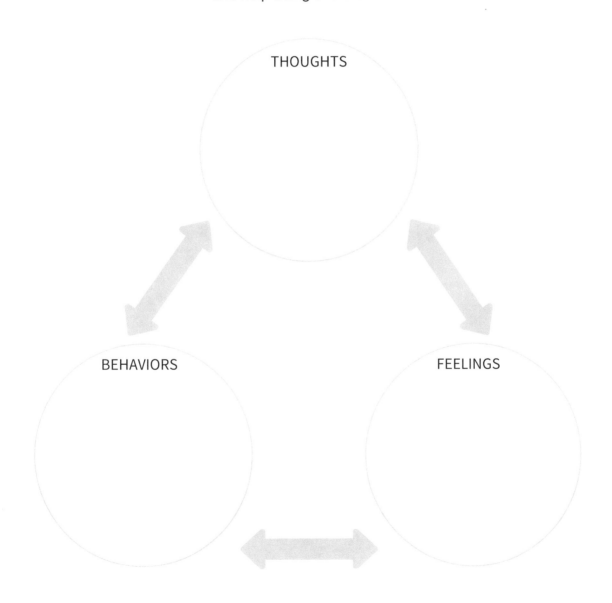

THOUGHTS

BEHAVIORS

FEELINGS

Thoughts / Feelings / Behaviors Triangle

This is a tool that may help you start to make sense of what causes your feelings.
Please seek the guidance of a licensed mental health professional if you would like help using this tool.

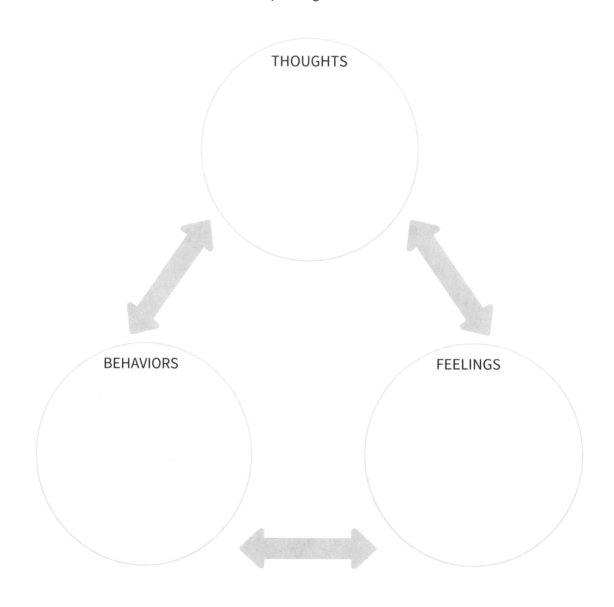

THOUGHTS

BEHAVIORS

FEELINGS

Cognitive Reframing

This is a technique that may help you modify your Thoughts/Feelings/Behaviors pattern.
Please seek the guidance of a licensed mental health professional if you would like help using this technique.

SITUATION
a short description of what happened - only the facts

MY ACTUAL THOUGHT	ALTERNATE THOUGHT

THOUGHTS
interpret the situation using your thoughts (note that interpretations are not always accurate - there are many ways to think about the same situation)

FEELINGS
identify the feelings you experience as a result of your actual thought - and the ones you may have with the alternate thought (you can use the Feelings Wheel to help with this)

BEHAVIOR
decide how you will use, cope with or express your feelings - do this for the feelings connected to your actual thought and your alternate thought

Cognitive Reframing

This is a technique that may help you modify your Thoughts/Feelings/Behaviors pattern.
Please seek the guidance of a licensed mental health professional if you would like help using this technique.

SITUATION
a short description of what happened - only the facts

	MY ACTUAL THOUGHT	ALTERNATE THOUGHT
THOUGHTS interpret the situation using your thoughts (note that interpretations are not always accurate - there are many ways to think about the same situation)		
FEELINGS identify the feelings you experience as a result of your actual thought - and the ones you may have with the alternate thought (you can use the Feelings Wheel to help with this)		
BEHAVIOR decide how you will use, cope with or express your feelings - do this for the feelings connected to your actual thought and your alternate thought		

Cognitive Reframing

This is a technique that may help you modify your Thoughts/Feelings/Behaviors pattern.
Please seek the guidance of a licensed mental health professional if you would like help using this technique.

SITUATION
a short description of what happened - only the facts

	MY ACTUAL THOUGHT	ALTERNATE THOUGHT
THOUGHTS interpret the situation using your thoughts (note that interpretations are not always accurate - there are many ways to think about the same situation)		
FEELINGS identify the feelings you experience as a result of your actual thought - and the ones you may have with the alternate thought (you can use the Feelings Wheel to help with this)		
BEHAVIOR decide how you will use, cope with or express your feelings - do this for the feelings connected to your actual thought and your alternate thought		

Cognitive Reframing

This is a technique that may help you modify your Thoughts/Feelings/Behaviors pattern.
Please seek the guidance of a licensed mental health professional if you would like help using this technique.

SITUATION

a short description of what happened - only the facts

MY ACTUAL THOUGHT	ALTERNATE THOUGHT

THOUGHTS

interpret the situation using your thoughts (note that interpretations are not always accurate - there are many ways to think about the same situation)

FEELINGS

identify the feelings you experience as a result of your actual thought - and the ones you may have with the alternate thought (you can use the Feelings Wheel to help with this)

BEHAVIOR

decide how you will use, cope with or express your feelings - do this for the feelings connected to your actual thought and your alternate thought

Cognitive Reframing

This is a technique that may help you modify your Thoughts/Feelings/Behaviors pattern.
Please seek the guidance of a licensed mental health professional if you would like help using this technique.

SITUATION
a short description of what happened - only the facts

MY ACTUAL THOUGHT	ALTERNATE THOUGHT

THOUGHTS
interpret the situation using your thoughts (note that interpretations are not always accurate - there are many ways to think about the same situation)

FEELINGS
identify the feelings you experience as a result of your actual thought - and the ones you may have with the alternate thought (you can use the Feelings Wheel to help with this)

BEHAVIOR
decide how you will use, cope with or express your feelings - do this for the feelings connected to your actual thought and your alternate thought

Coping With Feelings

Write a list of your favorite actions that help you cope with challenging feelings.
(It's also okay to include things you haven't done yet but want to try!)

Notes About My Feelings

Made in the USA
Columbia, SC
23 February 2025

54160262R00080